R·EVOLUTION

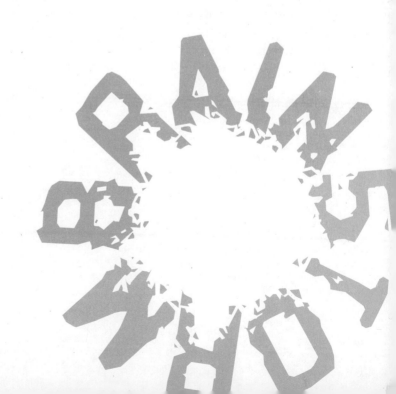

R·EVOLUTION

true mental health stories
of love, personal evolution,
and cultural revolution

HEATHER DOWN • NATALIE HARRIS • COURTNEY TAYLOR

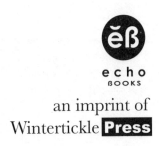

ĕß

echo
BOOKS

an imprint of
Wintertickle Press

Library and Archives Canada Cataloguing in Publication

Down, Heather, 1966-, author
    Brainstorm revolution : true mental health stories of love, personal evolution, and cultural revolution / Heather Down, Natalie Harris, Courtney Taylor.

ISBN 978-1-894813-95-2 (softcover)

    1. Mentally ill--Social networks. 2. Interpersonal relations. 3. Love. 4. Self-actualization (Psychology). 5. Mentally ill--Social life and customs. 6. Mental illness--Social aspects. 7. Mentally ill--Biography. I. Harris, Natalie M., author II. Taylor, Courtney, 1983-, author III. Title.

RA790.5.D696 2018   616.890092'2   C2018-904452-7

PRINTED IN CANADA

Published by Wintertickle Press
132 Commerce Park Drive, Unit K, Suite 155, Barrie, ON, L4N 0Z7
winterticklepress.com

My friends, love is better than anger.
Hope is better than fear. Optimism is better
than despair. So let us be loving, hopeful, and
optimistic. And we'll change the world.

– Jack Layton

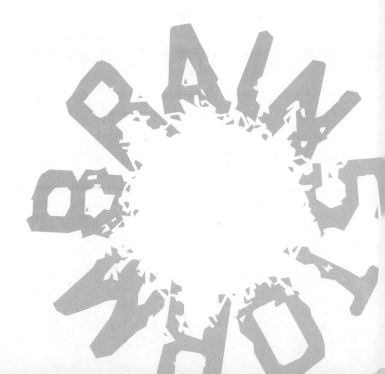

CONTENT & TRIGGER WARNING

The content of this book will include discussion and description of mental health and illness experiences that may be difficult and/or triggering for some. Some topics may include, but are not limited to, abuse (physical, mental, emotional, verbal, sexual); child abuse; self-injurious behavior (self-harm, eating disorders, etc.); suicide; death or dying; pregnancy/childbirth; miscarriages; violent crime/home invasions; description of war; and mental illness.

CONTENTS

PART II: EVOLUTION - 77

PART III: REVOLUTION - 167

FOREWORD

It's hard to see things clearly in the dark.
— Zoey Raffay, "Calling for Me," p. 146

I ALMOST QUIT.

I was just about done with mental health advocacy. I was done with the school assemblies. I was done with the conferences. I was done with the interviews and media appearances. I was done with the community events, the support groups, the volunteering, the town halls, the meetings with politicians, the earnest pleas for reform. And I was especially done with the thing that has had the most impact in my mental health advocacy life—I was done with public speaking. I had decided that I was going to finish up the projects I was working on, and then I would quit championing for mental health altogether. I wasn't sure what I would do afterward—maybe I'd pursue one of my childhood ambitions and become a software engineer or perhaps a sports journalist. I don't know. All I knew was that I didn't want to do this mental health crusading thing anymore.

And then I was presented with the opportunity: the honour and the invitation to provide the foreword for this book. As ambivalent as I was about my future in advocacy, I still thought I'd give this foreword thing a shot because, after all, I'm a guy who likes parties, and I never turn down an invitation. God, am I glad that I didn't turn down this one.

> I realize that the pain I have withstood when held
> in its maddening grip has been transformed into a
> weapon I can yield to save others from its suffocation.
> – Courtney Taylor, "In the Dark of Night," p. 69

But before I start talking about this incredible collection of stories, let's press rewind for a minute—I want to explain how my connection to this work came to be.

To put it bluntly, I come from tragedy.

There is a history of physical, emotional, and sexual abuse in my family that goes back generations. My grandmother was a victim of such abuse, as were most of her eight children, my mother being the oldest of the lot. Instability dominated my mother's existence as she moved dozens of times throughout her upbringing, scrounging through shantytown refuse for food, having to fight for her life—literally—on more than one occasion. My father, on the other hand, was neglected and ridiculed by family and community alike because of a stutter that persisted throughout his childhood and youth. Yes, my homeland of Jamaica is a beautiful country, but it's a hard country, plagued by poverty and a shockingly high murder rate, derived from political corruption ruthlessly enforced by street gangs. These are the main reasons why my parents brought my brothers and me to Toronto, Canada.

I was almost three years old, my brothers nine and ten. My parents were still married. Then they split. My mom, my brothers, and I ended up living in a shelter until we were able to move out into public housing. Unfortunately, there was a white su-premacist gang in that building that tried their best to terrorize us. When my father threatened my mom's life, we moved two weeks before I started high school. BOOM—friends gone. When my mom became suicidal and had a psychotic break, I quickly forgot what happiness and excitement felt like. I stopped leaving the house or socializing. Depression and anxiety took over. We were poor, and I resorted to petty crime to feed myself. My mom improved but I didn't. Three suicide notes and several ER visits later, I found myself on Lorazepam and in counselling. I improved; I graduated with an undergraduate degree; I got a job and a girlfriend. I was ready to move on from my mental health story.

Then I was asked—well, more like volun-told—to tell my story at a youth mental health conference. In my head, I could only imagine the snickers, the derision, the judgment, and the rejection I'd receive from these teenagers. I didn't want to do it, but I did it anyway. And instead of laughing *at* me, they laughed *with* me. Instead of being bored to tears, they were moved to tears by my story. Since then, I've told my story hundreds of times to tens of thousands of people. My story has opened doors. It has taken me all over the world, and it has led me to my wife. It has put me in documentaries, on TV, on radio, and plastered my likeness like a mural all over the virtual walls of the Internet. Hell, in the past year my story has given me two TEDx talks and national recognition as a CAMH 150 Difference Maker for my contributions to mental health advocacy in Canada. Just three months ago, I was a co-emcee at an event with the former VP of Twitter, eating lunch with Jim Treliving of *Dragon's Den* and Boston Pizza fame, and getting hugs from the prime minister's mother. This is all incredible stuff, but the biggest gift that telling my story has given me has been the incredible people I've met. I now have something I never had growing up, and that's a community of open-minded, compassionate, sensitive people who see me and accept me for all who I am.

And yet, just two weeks ago, I was ready to give it all up. I was tired of being so open. I was also scared of being vulnerable for the first time since I started my advocacy journey at that youth mental health conference almost eight years ago. I was unsure that my authenticity was being properly appreciated. I was being jerked around by event organizers, some folks not honouring payment agreements, and generally being treated like some sort of social justice mercenary rather than a person. This made me feel like the emotional skydive I take every time I tell my story wasn't at all valued.

Enter Courtney Taylor from stage left, bringing with her the opportunity to share these words, but more importantly, the opportunity to read this book.

> I have discovered that the most impactful thing
> I can do is simply talk about my experiences.
> – Michael Landsberg, "Do You Want Dinner?" p. 215

This book is an absolute triumph. As I write this, I'm shaking my head, trying to move past the emotional wall of awe-inspired incredulity I'm experiencing, as I attempt to come up with some arrangement of words that can approach a modicum of accuracy in describing the revolutionary power of the stories you are about to read.

The stories held herein are nothing less than life-changing.

These stories are diverse, authored by real everyday people who, like all of us, have lived ordinarily extraordinary lives. Most of the contributors are not famous. These stories come from the mother with family in tow in the grocery store and the son whose bike is the most important thing in the world to him. These are not just mental health stories. These are real-life stories. These are stories of loss, happiness, pain, addiction, recovery, illness, discovery, humour, irony, serendipity, growth, learning, and forgiveness. These are stories of evolution, revolution, and love.

I know that you, the reader, will enjoy these stories as much as I did. You will absorb them, and they will coalesce in your soul, coming to live inside of you, changing your perspective of your own experiences. Perhaps you'll be moved to tears countless times like I was, compelled by the strength and resiliency of these writers. Perhaps these stories will reinvigorate you and provide you with the motivation and courage to tell your own story for the first time, or to tell it again—like it has done for me. What I do know for sure is this book will draw you in like a riptide, and you won't want to escape.

Thank you, Courtney, for reaching out to me with this opportunity. Thank you, Heather, for your patience and for entrusting me with this section of the book. Thank you to everyone else who contributed to this dazzling work of art—to those I know and to those I don't. All of these stories are valuable. All of these stories are awesome. Thank you most of all to you, the reader, who, by reading these stories and sharing them, will bring them to life and help drive the Brainstorm Revolution forward.

I just keep going.
– Enza Tiberi-Checchia, "The Question," p. 218

As for me, this book has given me life again as an advocate, and I will continue to approach this work with passion, compassion, optimism, and hope. I will continue telling my story. Now, reader, I speak directly to you once more with one simple request—let's walk this journey together.

Asante Haughton

ACKNOWLEDGEMENTS

Wintertickle Press would like to acknowledge the financial contributions to help make this project possible from Christie Bond, Jake Forsyth, Tim Grutzius, Ryan Knight, Amber Phillips, Deb Snow, Enza Tiberi-Checchia, and Connie Watson.

ABBREVIATIONS

ADHD	attention deficit hyperactivity disorder
CAMH	Centre of Addiction and Mental Health
CBC	Canadian Broadcasting Corporation
CD	Canadian Forces Decoration
CM	Member of the Order of Canada
CMHA	Canadian Mental Health Association
EAL	equine assisted learning
ECG	electrocardiogram
LGBTQ	lesbian, gay, bisexual, transgender, queer
MHI	Mental Health Innovations (company)
MP	Minister of Parliament
MRI	magnetic resonance imaging
MS	multiple sclerosis
MSC	Meritorious Service Cross
OCD	obsessive-compulsive disorder
OSI	operational stress injury
PTSD	post-traumatic stress disorder
TSN	The Sports Network

INTRODUCTION
Courtney Taylor

NOT EVEN TWELVE HOURS BEFORE writing these words, I was talking with my friend Natalie Harris, hoarding her generous support while experiencing a spike in my usually well-managed anxiety.

My anxiety. I suppose that's where all of this began for me.

As a child, I suffered from multiple phobias, intense sleep disturbances, and severe separation anxiety, causing me to miss out on common childhood activities such as sleepovers and class trips. Though I didn't know how to name them at the time, I experienced panic attacks and would often run home from school shortly after the first bell rang, before even stepping into class. I suffered from stomach aches daily and was put through a series of physical tests. I was placed on a lactose-free diet, as doctors guessed at a diagnosis to cure what ailed me. But nothing changed. All through my childhood, my "nervousness" contin-ued, plaguing me with worry and the constant awareness that I was not the same as all my friends.

Eventually, at seven years old, after a psychiatric consulta-tion, I was diagnosed with an anxiety disorder.

As I entered my teenage years, my panic attacks increased and intensified, and it was then that one of the multiple psychiatrists, psychologists, or social workers I had seen in the years since my diagnosis recommended medication. I started taking a common antidepressant when I was thirteen years old.

Now, slightly over twenty years later, I'm writing an introduction for a book that features an inspiring collection of mental health stories. My own story brought me to this point, first leading me down a path of advocacy in 2013. Since then, I've learned, powerfully, that sharing saves lives. I've been granted tremendous opportunities, from meeting fellow change makers I respect and admire to sharing my voice in articles that have reached thousands. I've had the privilege of comforting others as they cried over loss, and I've witnessed years of debilitating shame and silence fall away from people. Gratefully, in my own moments of darkness, I've also had many allies to count on, lean on, and help me through.

As I write this, I'm coming out of a (thankfully) short bout of depression brought on by a severe spike in my anxiety. It is not lost on me that a woman I had not met even a year ago is one of the many I'm fortunate to have offering me support, love, and a shoulder to lean on.

Natalie and I originally connected on social media, not meeting in person until August 2017. At one of the handful of events we both attended, Natalie was accompanied by her friend Heather Down of Wintertickle Press, who suggested we work together to create the book you're holding right now. Less than a year later, that quick, enthusiastic conversation is now a tangible reality. It has been brought to life by those who contributed so boldly and by three people who were connected by nothing more than their shared passion for a cause and their own lived experiences.

The page you're reading right now, and the many others that follow, stamped with honesty and bravery, are what can come from sharing. When we open up about our mental health struggles, share our stories without shame, something like this book can be the outcome. That beautiful knowledge leaves me speechless.

The stigma of mental health, though improved, is still alive and well. But with every new admission of an experience or a battle that one might feel they sit in alone, another brick is added onto the house of support we're building together. Held in the warmth and comfort of one another, bound by our similar narratives, we feel like we've found a home.

Sharing the darkest moments of my life has made my life. I know that my journey will not always be easy, but I also know that when it gets hard, I never stand alone. I am surrounded by a community of others who understand every tormented thought and wretched emotion I've ever had. The proof is in these pages.

But make no mistake, this book isn't written just for those who personally experience mental illness and their allies. The universal themes of courage, personal realization, and social change apply to all humankind. And to truly make lasting cultural shifts, talking only among ourselves, comfortably in our own labelled boxes, isn't going to work. We all need to reach a little farther. In order for us all to understand each other, we need to communicate—and do so beyond our personal borders.

This book is divided into three parts: Love, Evolution, and Revolution. Initially, in the development of this project, the first section was Revolution. During the review of the book, several members of a focus group suggested that the book may be too "heavy." "But it gets lighter as the book goes on," Heather explained to them. One member replied, "But what good is that if the reader puts it down before they get there?"

After much thought, Heather contacted me. And what she said to both Natalie and me was profound. "The answer to the book is the answer to *everything:* Always start with love."

PART I

LOVE

love
[ləv]

concern for the good of another

a benevolent, compassionate kindness: to wish
the best for someone

THE STORM

V.N. Doran

FOR TEN YEARS I'VE TRIED to beat back the nebulous black. I've looked at knives the way that people look at God. Sun on the blade, blade in the hand, blade on the skin, hot and holy and serene. I thought that maybe I could bleed the crazy out, let just enough of that summertime blood go singing down the drain. Not enough to end up in the underneath, just enough to purge and purify. Just enough to reset the synapses and leave my body innocent and clean. But I'm a coward. So instead I tried to starve the crazy out. I let hunger reach long hands into that deep and awful black. But when hunger created another shell of pain around the pain, I tried to drown it out with carbs and crap and alcohol. But the black is still there, always there, staining the edges, swelling under my eyes, catching in my throat, splitting my pelvis with its teratoid tongue.

Today an ice storm rages, and it is the first time the outside world resembles the inside of my head. I drive to the car factory for my shift through a deluge of freezing rain, my wipers squealing against the glass, barely keeping up. When I arrive at work, I have to glide over the parking lot, bent forward and shuffling like a penguin, to keep myself from falling on the newly frosted ground. The rain splatters heavily against my hood and my sleeves and my chest and my boots, dotting my winter clothes with crystalline petals that don't melt until I get inside the building. I pull out my phone to find a text message from my love: Please drive safely and let me know when you've arrived! I smile and send a quick response.

The factory, with its vast metallic light, its fluorescence and its plastic and its grey, its robots, its many uniformed men and its countless, countless skeletons of half-built cars, blocks out everything else that exists.

I change into my uniform in the locker room, shivering under the thin white fabric, then make my way to my place on the line: Zone 8. There are no windows near the line, and the ceilings arch so high above that there is no way to hear the brutal teeth of the rain. My colleagues and I gather near the team leader's desk to listen to the daily meeting.

"So far everything is running smoothly. We should have a normal shift, as far as I know, but of course that could change," my team leader, Derek, says, shuffling his papers. I hear someone behind me snicker and complain.

"I can't believe they made us drive in for this shit. Guarantee you they'll send us home early and we'll have to drive back through this mess in the damn dark." The bell rings and we disperse to our various stations.

Derek is right; for a time, the shift proceeds normally. I drill in brake bolts and door strikers and bumper spacers, checking torques, doing up couplers, my knuckles aching, forearms burning, sweat making the back of my shirt cling. I've done these jobs thousands upon thousands of times. My body knows how to move without my brain. And that leaves my brain in a dangerous place. There is nothing to distract when on the line. The black pulses at the edges, stretches itself out, an ominous thrum infiltrating bone and sinew, spurred on by the movement of my limbs, transforming into rage. I throw my gun more heavily than I should into one of the bins at my station, scattering bolts, then hear someone nearby remark, "Damn. Everybody seems so pissed off today." The comment makes me want to take up my gun again and plunge it directly into my right eye. But then I may have trouble getting home. I will need both eyes to see through the darkness of the storm.

As the line chugs along to its monotonous rhythm, sending cars forward through the dust, I try to batten down the bleeding of the black. I think about my love. He would be home from work by now. I picture him coming through the front door of our house, petting our two cats, and calling out a greeting, as if I were there. I take a step forward, reaching for him, casting my mind out over the storm-torn ground to find him. I press my body up against his, feel the sturdy warmth of him penetrate, feel his hands move up over my back. As I open my mouth to speak to him, I blink, brought back to myself. I have fallen behind. I run back to the car that has just passed me by, frantically grabbing for my gun while Derek laughs at me and asks, "Ronnie, do you need help?"

Do I need help?

I asked myself such a thing before. And I turned to the rigours of medical love and its twin therapies: meditation and medication. Meditation made time stretch out and disappear so fast that it took my breath with it. Medication made me euphoric, with heart palpitations that soon turned to nausea.

They both made my brain feel fizzy yet flat, dull yet sparked with a desperate half-light. The only therapy that really seemed to make a difference was being with my love. The first time I cried in front of him, I felt ashamed. Now I cry in front of him almost daily. When he tries to ask what's wrong, I have no answer. Any wrongness comes from within my own body, and there is no reason and no cure. When he asks me what to do, I say, "Just stay here, like this." He holds me in the shuddering of the night, holding my hands, holding my heart. Holding my body together.

The line jerks to a stop. I, too, stop and wait, wondering if things will start back up again. I glance at the clock: 9:18 p.m. Three hours to go. I walk to a nearby car and sit in the gaping hole of the door frame, settling into the space where the driver's seat will eventually be installed. Suddenly cheering erupts over the plant, broken up by shouts of "see you, boys!" and "home time!" I stand, trying to make sense of the scene. Derek jogs up to me, putting his walkie-talkie back into his pocket as he nears.

"The company across the street that supplies our parts lost power and we can't get any more. We're shutting down now. Thanks for coming in tonight, Ronnie."

I nod my understanding, and as he turns to walk away, he pauses.

"Be safe out there."

The words are apt. When I emerge from the building, I don't recognize the outside world. The ice has more than doubled and everything is strange and thick and silver under the streetlights. Trees have been turned to glass, their branches heavy with the weight of their dangerous beauty. The cars in the lot are totally encased in ice, and I hear the sharp cracking of scrapers against windows and doors. When I reach my own car after a treacherous walk, it takes more than fifteen minutes to break through the cold calluses the rain has left there. I pull out of the parking lot ten times more slowly than I normally do and feel panic rise in my chest as my car, a reliable Toyota Corolla, struggles to respond to my commands.

Things only get worse out on the roads. I leave the factory later than everyone else, and I am almost completely alone as I drive. My fingers grip the steering wheel tighter than they gripped the bolts and guns at work. My throat feels dry as I lean forward in my seat, staring out over the alien landscape through the onslaught of the rain. Ahead, I see a police car parked lengthwise across the road, lights flashing, red warnings in the night. A downed tree blocks the way just behind the cruiser, crackling and corpse-like. After a few moments, I manage to get myself turned around and embark on a different path just as the ice bites down on power lines overhead. Sparks explode, arcing in a fiery spray, turning the silver of the scene to burnished magma.

More downed trees make me backtrack again. And again. And still the rain falls, and lightning tears up the sky, and thunder threatens to crack the world in two. But I recognize something in the storm. Through the animal fear, I latch onto a familiar feeling. The wind with its wordless scream, the painful gashes of light erupting, the cold so big it breaks my heart, the ice so slick it is malicious—they echo the mechanisms of my own mind. The great throbbing of the earth under the storm reminds me of my body faltering under the burden of the black. I pull over to the side of the road, turning off the engine. I am running out of gas. I wonder if it would be better to lean into the darkness, to let the storm take my body down, to let that deeply familiar pain clasp onto me and synthesize. Driving is so difficult tonight. It would be easy to remain, then disappear.

I glance at my phone. The battery has been drained. The clock tells me I have been driving for almost ninety minutes. Normally it takes less than thirty to get home from the factory.

While looking at my phone, I notice multiple messages from my love, asking me how I am, where I am, when I will get home, if I am safe. In this moment, I know that I can never let this go, can never let the blackness take me from my love. My love is the lighthouse, the landmark, the beacon on the shore, reaching illuminated arms toward me, guiding me home.

I start up the car again, easing back out onto the road. The wind and the rain and the ice and the dark fight me every step of the way, howling, trying to pull me back. But slowly, slowly and steadily, I orient myself, preparing myself for one last drive, one last shot to make it back. The storm can tear at me on all sides, but I have a car with snow tires and a warm coat and good boots and a beautiful love waiting for me on the other side, beckoning. I can see him there, waiting, where he will always wait, just past the point of irreparable wounds, past the thorns and the sorrows and the edges of the black. And I know that I will always go to him.

In the morning, after the storm, I wake up safe beside my love. I lean against him, observing the magnificent world as it glistens, luminous with the history of its pain.

V.N. Doran holds a master's degree in creative writing from the University of Toronto. She is the recipient of the Maureen Morgan English Award and the Avie Bennett Emerging Writer's Award. She has published both poetry and prose in anthologies like *Lake Effect 6* as well as in magazines like *The Northern Appeal* and *Petal Journal.* She currently lives in Barrie, Ontario, with her partner and two cats and is finishing her first novel.

THREE AND CHANGE

Glen Oliver

I STOP AT THE SAME drive-thru at a nearby coffee shop almost every morning on my way to work. It is a sunny July day. "I'll have a large coffee with half a milk, please," I speak into the intercom.

"Is that all?" the faceless voice booms back at me through the teakettle-grey metal box.

"Yes," I reply.

I wait as the cars creep up to the window so their drivers can receive paper cups of hot coffee and brown bags of morning treats.

I get to the window and see the familiar sight of the server.

"Hi Glen. That'll be one dollar and ninety-five cents."

"Oh wait," I hesitate. Once or twice a week, I've been in the habit of paying the bill for the car behind me. "How much for the next order?" I ask.

"Three and change. They ordered a coffee and a muffin."

"Add that to my bill, please," I instruct.

"No problem."

"And remember to say, 'Have a great day' when you tell them it's been paid for."

I always ask the server to remind the recipient to "Have a great day." It's my thing.

I pay my bill, grab my coffee, and drive off to work where I am a property manager, hardly giving the morning events a second thought.

Days melt into weeks, and weeks ripple into months—the coffee and muffin incident fades, resting just beneath recent memories.

My wife, Linda, and I have four grown children, and our lives have shifted from the busyness and hectic schedules of raising a young family to a more steady, pleasant rhythm of comfortable work and home-life balance. Days are fuelled by routine, shopping, errands, time together, playing tennis, and entertaining friends and family.

One habit Linda has is to scour the local newspaper, sifting through flyers and coupons in preparation for our shopping trips. I have learned to ask first before chucking the paper into the recycle bin in case I have accidentally thrown out the "deal of the week."

I didn't sleep much the night before. It is a crisp Canadian November day and the only thing on my mind is taking a nap. I sprawl out on the longest side of our sectional to drift off while Linda busies herself by looking through the paper like a miner panning for gold. It doesn't take long until I am asleep.

The pure joy of a midday nap is short-lived, however. I am awakened to the sound of crying.

At first I wonder if I am dreaming, but I am not. What could it be? Linda wouldn't be crying over a missed sale on canned peaches.

"What is it?" I ask, blinking my eyes partially open.

"You have to read this," she says, pointing at a page in the local paper.

"I don't have my reading glasses. I will read it later," I mumble as I roll over, hoping to fall back to sleep.

She is still crying. Her tone changes. "Read this now." She stands up, and her comment feels like more of a directive than a suggestion.

I sigh. "I can't see."

This does not deter her. With a slight annoyance, she locates my reading glasses on the end table, hands them to me, and repeats, still crying, "Read this . . . *now.*"

I put on my glasses, straighten out the crinkly paper with a snap, and look at the article she is pointing to.

It is an article about a letter that was sent to the paper. I start to read, "I had planned to end it all at home in my own little ritual and explain my thoughts in a note for anyone who cares."

What is this? Why does Linda want me to read it?

Then the lightbulb turns on. The article continues to say that on July 18, the author of the letter was planning to die. He—or she—had written a note and then went to the drive-thru of a nearby coffee shop at the corner of Kingston and Glendale to order a coffee and a muffin. Upon arriving at the window, the author learned that the man in the SUV had already paid.

"That man in the SUV is me," I say, dumbfounded.

Linda nods.

I feel my eyes well up as I read on. "The nice man already paid for it and he said to have a great day."

"I wondered why someone would buy coffee for a stranger for no reason. Why me? Why today? If I was a religious sort,

I would take this as a sign. This random act of kindness was directed at me on this day for a purpose.

"I decided at that moment to change my plans for the day and do something nice for someone. I ended up helping a neighbour take groceries out of her car and into the house.

"To the nice man in the SUV . . . thank you from the bottom of my heart, and know your kind gesture has truly saved a life."

It was only three dollars and change. But sometimes the smallest gesture can make the biggest difference in someone's life.

I look at my wife before reading the next line: "On July 18, 2017, I not only had a great day, I had the *greatest* day!"

Sometimes folks ask me if I ever think about the people for whom I buy a coffee. I answer, "I do now!" I can't help but think that if everyone showed a little more kindness now and then, the world would be a better place.

Glen Oliver works in property management in Toronto, Ontario. This father of four adult children believes that kindness is the answer to many questions.

BIRTH OF A FIRST RESPONDER

April Shaw

PARAMEDICS, FIREFIGHTERS, AND POLICE OFFICERS all have something in common. When crisis arrives and everyone's running away from it, they're the ones running toward it. They're the first on the scene to help, to rescue, and to serve. In my world, the term "first responder" means something a little different.

The first year after my son's autism diagnosis was by far the hardest. The news hit us like a Mack truck. We were lost, confused, and in many ways in a state of grieving what could've been. But probably more than anything, I felt alone. I'll never forget our initial first responder, Dana. She was the first one to reach out. She had a son with autism, and she told us that the first year would be the roughest, but she also told us things would get better. She said we'd find our therapists (we did). She said we'd find a school (we did). She said we'd find our village (we did). She said we'd find our way (we did). She was the first of our first responders.

Spring has sprung, and the weather is getting warm again. We live in an apartment with a community pool, and we venture out early to avoid the extreme heat, the crowds, and to be honest, yes, the stares. One time a gentleman (term used loosely here), after looking at my son, motioned to his wife that circular motion between his ear and head. You know, the one people use to indicate someone's crazy. Yeah, that happened. People aren't always kind. That day, as we walked back toward the apartment, I contemplated all the things I could've and should've said. And I may have possibly considered running him over with my Prius. Okay, maybe not run over, but at least tap him with my front bumper. (That'll teach him!) But instead of doing any of that, I went home and I cried, and then I cried some more. I avoided the pool after that as much as I could. My son stims—and he stims a lot. Finger-flicking, hand-flapping, and squealing. Behaviour that makes him appear weird to some people. Kids rarely initiate play with him, and typically when they do, as soon as they realize he's different, they walk away. They always walk away.

Except today . . .

I am sitting by the pool, watching my son splash and squeal, doing his stimmy thing, happy as a clam. In walks Jade, somewhere between seven and eight years old, blond hair, freckles across her nose, all fifty pounds of her, if that. She notices he is by himself and proceeds to initiate play. She talks, asks him questions, and as usual he doesn't respond. About this time, I fully expect her to walk away just like all the others have before her, but she doesn't. She doesn't walk away. Instead, she looks at me and asks, "Does he talk?"

I respond, "No, he does not."

She asks, "Does he have autism?"

I'm not going to lie here, the question stuns me a little. I am not entirely sure how to explain autism to a girl so young. Either way, my response is short and simple. "Yes, he does."

She turns around and changes her approach with him. Instead of asking him questions, she starts telling him what to do. "Here, get on the float. I'll pull you. I'll throw the ball and you catch, okay?"

Whoa! Am I really seeing what I am seeing? Is my son playing? Does my son finally have a friend? For about twenty minutes, until the little girl has to go, I watch two kids laughing and playing together, and, for the first time ever, one of them is mine. Thank goodness I have sunglasses on, because I am a mess. A blubbery, emotional mess at what I have just witnessed.

Had I not ventured back to the pool because I was too scared to have another encounter like the one with the "gentleman," I would've missed out on two remarkable things. The first one was this: In about twenty minutes, a little girl named Jade gave me something I'd waited six years to see. My son, *mine*, play with a friend! And the second thing I witnessed, well, that was equally remarkable: That warm summer day, I got to see a first responder being born. And that, my friends, is something you never forget.

April Shaw lives in Mobile, Alabama. She is a forty-three-year-old single mother of two. Her firstborn is a daughter named Raven, twenty-three, and her second is a son named Deuce, ten, who has severe nonverbal autism. Deuce uses an iPad for the majority of his communication.

CHANGING THE FRAME

Amber Phillips

"WHY ME?" I KEEP ASKING myself over and over again. I am over-thinking everything, right down to whether I am going to get out of bed this morning. I visualize myself as a cartoon character, running on a treadmill, out of control, unable to get off even if I want to. I wish it would just stop. I can't make sense of anything. I am physically and emotionally exhausted.

I feel my apartment walls closing in on me, and I know if I don't do something, a panic attack will take hold. I need air and I need it quickly. I force myself out of bed, throw on some clothes, and head to the nearby beach for a walk.

As I head out the door, my body feels sandwiched between the dull, drab grey sky glaring down on me and the dismal slate-coloured sidewalk crying up to me. I pass a man. "Good morning," he offers. "Good morning," I counter, more mono-tone than I wish.

When I get to the beach, the powdery leaden neutrality of the sand permeates my mind. I take off my sandals and feel the tepid granules between my toes: warm—but not warm enough. The sombre wind dances on my face: not quite a cele-bration. I look out at the dull, crashing waves and the gloomy, silvery sky. "Why me?" I ask again, aloud and alone, my mood matching every single flat hue and tone of grey my eyes can perceive.

A week passes, and I decide to take another walk along the beach. Just about out the door, I notice my Nikon sitting on the table. It is an impulse decision; I reach over and grab my old friend. "Hey, I'll bring you along today." I speak to this inanimate object as if it has the ability to hear me.

"Good morning," a young woman pushing a stroller says to me.

"Good morning," I answer, inflections inadvertently escaping through my voice. "How are you today?" I hear myself say.

At first, my muscles feel like they are coiled up like a spring. I snap a few shots of the water and notice I am starting to relax. I feel safe behind the lens, like my camera gives me superpowers and shields me from people's judgments, criticisms, stares, and the outside world itself.

I find a scene that looks good in the frame of my camera. I select the mode and I focus, taking a deep breath and snapping the picture, knowing I am truly living in the moment.

The texture of the sand, the vivid feathers on the soaring eagle, the kaleidoscope of iridescent shades in the water, the exquisite and varied tones in the sky, the resplendent beauty of all the nature around me—it all takes my breath away. I am in awe and escape my own head, focusing on the things around me. The world becomes sumptuous and colourful. The need to ruminate *Why me?* lessens.

I feel a calmness in my mind and body that I haven't felt in years. With photography, it is just me, my camera, and the nature in my lens. I love it and it loves me back. With the discovery of this new frame, it is just me (and me alone) who must take responsibility for my actions and decisions. It is a choice and a perspective I must choose—and this is the picture I wish to take every day from now on.

Amber Phillips is a photographer and writer. She resides in the shoreline town of Southampton, Ontario. She loves to read memoirs, thrillers, and true-to-life stories. She is excited to live life now and has no regrets about taking a leap of faith to change for the better. Looking for the perfect quote on the Internet, Amber realized there wasn't one that encapsulated how she truly felt, so she made her own: "I came to the realization that taking photographs is not just about getting the perfect shot. It is about capturing a moment in time that I get back and then I can cherish that photograph, knowing I truly lived in that moment."

MOTHER-DAUGHTER DRESSES

Deb McGrath

"I AM A TRANS WOMAN, I would like she-her pronouns, and my name is Hannah."

This is the sentence my son blurts out to me over the phone. Despite the bluntness of the statement, it isn't callous, ill-timed, or even cruel on his part. Truth be told, I have actually forced this on him. He has called to tell me he has something to say to me of utmost importance. He wants to talk to his dad and me at the same time, and his dad is out of town. Given the fact that I possess a particular and serious panic strain in my genetic makeup, I find myself, well . . . panicking. Has my boy found a lump? Is he ill? Dying? Is he injured? I would be picturing him at this very moment lying in a ditch wearing dirty underwear if I weren't talking to him on the phone.

I conjure the mere thread of authority I have over my twenty-five-year-old and say, "No, you have to tell me now!"

"I would rather wait" is his measured response.

I can feel all the saliva I possess leaving my body for damper pastures. I cannot leave this hanging to save my life. So, I push and plead and cajole and beg. It is, I confess, a shameless display. Clearly, I am not above it.

After some more back-and-forth, he says, "I am a trans woman, I would like she-her pronouns, and my name is Hannah."

I pause to take it in, or at least lie to myself that I am taking it in, and then I blurt out in an upbeat fashion, "I am so happy for you. Very happy. And you know that your father and I will support you a hundred percent and it's wonderful and I'm not super surprised and you are such a wonderful person and we really don't care what you do with your life as long as . . ."

Dear God, I have to find a way to shut up. I am exhausting myself.

I like to think of myself as what I call "an emotional first responder." I hear information from someone I love, and I put on my support cape. Then I swoop in to distribute accolades, platitudes, and general support, willy-nilly. Breathe. Breathe. So I do. Then . . .

"So . . . ummm . . . why Hannah?" I hear myself say.

So there it is. Apparently, my takeaway from this huge life-changing moment is the name.

"Hannah" is my issue. Shallow waters run deep.

She responds in a very calm manner. "Mom, you know how much I loved Cheryl's dog."

"You are naming yourself after Hannah the dog? Really?"

She considers this and says, "I thought the name was soft and pretty, and I need my name to be soft and pretty. Does that make sense?"

Of course it makes sense. My heart aches with shame. I am officially a bad person.

So . . .

Because it has been a few minutes since I have launched into a panicked run-on sentence, I say, "Well if you love the name Hannah, I love the name Hannah and I am sure your father will love the name Hannah and I am so glad it makes you feel beautiful because you are beautiful inside and out and I support this choice a hundred percent. After all, honey, it's your life and you are old enough to make your own choices and . . ."

At this point I am desperately hoping someone will hand me a pill. Or failing the availability of a pill, simply stuff something into my mouth. Where is my husband when I need him?

Hannah cuts in to stop my runaway train by saying, "Thanks, Mom. I love you so much, and I knew you would support me. Why don't I come over the day Dad gets home, and we can have dinner and spend time talking?"

"Of course . . . yes . . . ummm . . . *Hannah* . . . we can do that. That would be great. What a wonderful idea . . . *Hannah*."

Mercifully, at this point she says, "Great. Love you. Bye."

Adding to my saliva-less state is a dearth of words and breath. She hangs up before I can respond.

I spend the next few hours pacing up and down stairs through our house, our two dogs at my heel. As I wrestle and sort the reasons I am upset, our dogs keep their firm focus on "Walk? Are we going for a walk?"

I have to really analyze my reaction and my feelings, and before long, it comes down to one thing. I am fine with it. Truly fine. I realize I am honestly not invested in my child's gender, just her humanity. My only issue in the end is fear. Fear for her safety, fear for how the world might treat her, fear for her heart.

Despite the calm reasoning, my next two nights of sleep are fraught with end-to-end nightmares. I do that thing where you try to stay awake for a while after you wake from a horrible nightmare so it doesn't follow you back into slumber. But these nightmares are in for the long haul.

I dream our son is lost. Our son is dead. We never had a son. I give birth, but when I look for my son, they tell me at the hospital that I am mistaken and that I had my appendix removed instead. Our son joins a tiny-house cult and is never heard from again.

And when I wake up, I am a walking zombie for the rest of the day, the bleak despair of those horrible dreams still clinging to me like possessed dryer sheets. The truth is I had made peace with the news and had no issues with the concept of her transition, but I am still deeply mourning the loss of our son. I didn't even get a chance to say goodbye.

She is a woman. And as much as I was prepared for it . . . I guess I just wasn't.

Also, in the light of this new day, I have to remind myself that this really shouldn't be a huge shock. A few years before she came out to us as transgender, she broke up with a girlfriend she had loved for four years. At that point, she told us she was bisexual and that she wanted to explore that. Then she began as she described "experimenting with my feminine side." Again, we were behind her. So, after almost a year of her slipping more feminine looks into her wardrobe, we became used to this new bi, fluid, femme, butch, male-female thing. It felt like she was rocking the whole alphabet with her identity. LGBTQ+ was left in the dust with this all-encompassing A to Z.

But then she lands.

Her dad comes home and gives my fragile state a little support. He is fine. No anxiety, no nightmares, just relaxed and accepting of the whole thing. Show-off! In the meantime, as a result of my deep and consistent anxiety, I resemble an eighty-year-old with dirty hair who had lived hard. Having no control over much else, I opt to shower. A good choice all round.

The day after my husband's return, we are in the kitchen preparing our daughter's favourite meal, awaiting her arrival. We are also busying ourselves as any parent would—practising pronouns. I am she-ing it up and her-ing it up, but I confess that every time I say "Hannah," it comes out reluctant and garbled like I am drunk and wearing my night guard.

The key turns in the door and in she-her walks. To my sweet shock and elation, no one is lost or missing. They are all here in the front hall. The *hes*, the *shes*, and the *thems*. All in one beautiful package. It is a stunning moment in our hearts. No one has left us. The same human we had first glimpsed twenty-five years ago is standing right in front of us. We all start to cry. Thank God it is all of us, as I am growing tired of being the overly emotional one.

We sit in our sunroom with wine in hand, and we talk. We talk all the talks there are to talk and ask all the questions that can be asked. We listen and we learn. During our chat, I make a mental note to head to the local bookstore to secure a volume of crib notes for pronouns, complete with definitions, if such a thing exists. The afternoon can only be described as an acronym-o-rama. As the conversation progresses and the questions become more detailed, my husband and I just want to learn more so we can respect and understand what our daughter is going through. We can see that she is exploring, too, not knowing exactly what her choices might be and taking her time to listen to her heart and to her mind.

Before long, the conversation evolves into our usual topics such as her work, her social life, and Japanese films. Suddenly, it is as if nothing has changed. And nothing has, really. Because there has always been just the three of us. We have enjoyed this tight little unit, and today is no different. It is the three of us again. Us and our beautiful girl. We eat her favourite meal, and then our lovely daughter goes home to her apartment.

We have months and months, slipping up on pronouns, and she is always patient, gently correcting us. We go out places with her, and people are mostly wonderful and supportive. Sure, she gets looks. She gets stares. She says she is fine with it. She says that people are just trying to figure her out.

A more generous soul than I am, I tell you.

Through everything, I am still stuck on the name. Lovely, yes, but not unique enough or powerful enough for this girl. But I realize that I have to let it go. In all honesty, I am grateful this is my only issue with her transition.

Then, in a surprise turn of events, she comes to us one day and says that many trans people come out with a name that they don't keep. She says she has been thinking about it and realizes she needs a name to hang her hat on, a coming-out name, if you will. She tells us she would love for us to be part of her new name process. She asks us to pitch her names from her Scottish-Irish background. I won't lie. I am elated and set to the task as soon as she is out of our sight. What a glorious thing to get to name her! I know it sounds silly, but it makes me feel like she is being born all over again.

It wasn't easy for me to get pregnant and despite hoping for two children, I could only have one. While we were expecting her, we didn't care if we had a boy or girl, but we hoped for one of each. Now we got our wish. We had a boy for twenty-five years, and we'll have a girl for the rest of our lives. I would rec- ommend that kind of labour to any woman.

After copious amounts of research, we present her with forty names. Her name now is officially Kinley, from the Irish side of our family. We all love it. Kin for short. It fits her. It belongs to her—and I am so proud to say, "She belongs to me."

It all *trans*pires beautifully until Kinley and I are out at a fair. A woman and her twenty-something daughter are nearby, and the daughter says to her mother, "There's a transvestite!" The mother wheels around and spews, "Where is it?"

It!

She says "it." I am gutted.

Their mouths agape, they look at us with such hate and such disgust that it leaves me breathless. The object of their ire is my lovely daughter.

I think I will expire right here on the spot as the daughter circles my daughter, looking her up and down as Kinley stands, frozen. We are stunned. As she walks away from my girl, I stumble over on rubber legs to this stranger and circle her the same way she has circled Kinley, looking her up and down, and then move close to her face and utter, "Uh huh," and walk away.

Trying to recover from this sickening moment, I say to Kinley, "This must make you so angry."

She says, "Mom, I can't afford to be angry. I just get frightened."

Frightened for just living your life? I think. *Frightened for existing?* I come home and tell my husband what has taken place and weep all my tears. After thinking about it, I realize that my response, although possibly warranted, was also aggressive and did not sit well with me. I decide to get some cards made so that, whenever it gets ugly, I can simply hand out one featuring a lovely pink flower on it that reads: MY DAUGHTER IS A TRANS WOMAN. SHE IS A LOVING AND KIND HUMAN BEING. PLEASE JOIN ME

IN SUPPORTING HER AND EVERY PERSON WHO IS TRYING TO LIVE THEIR AUTHENTIC LIFE. PEACE AND LOVE.

When the cards arrive in the mail, my husband laughs as I open the package of two hundred and fifty. "Wow, you're expecting trouble!" he says.

What can I tell you? There was a special on if you ordered that many.

A year passes, and I still have that full packet of two hundred and fifty cards. I am happy to say I haven't handed a single one out.

I have a daughter! That concept is burrowed in the sweet spot of my soul. I have a lovely, brave, poised, bright daughter. There should be a new word for pride. And our life as a trio continues as before. We share together old things like seeing films and new things like buying bras.

While clothes shopping today, we step out of the change room and we are both wearing the exact same dress. We laugh so hard, as it is easy to see the many layers in this pivotal moment. I buy the dress for me and treat Kinley to hers. At least that way I know she won't be raiding my closet!

Because that's what daughters do.

Deb McGrath has worked extensively in film, TV, and stage, including CBC's *Getting Along Famously*, which she created, wrote, and starred in with her husband, Colin Mochrie. *Little Mosque on the Prairie, The Ron James Show,* and most recently *Let's Get Physical* are just a few of the many series she has worked on. Deb has done numerous animated series and radio and TV voice spots, including being the voice of Winners for five years. Deb divides her creative time between writing screenplays and advocating for the LGBTQ community.

NOT NOW

Catherine Kenwell

I WAKE ON MY SIDE, curled up tight in a ball of skin and bone. Mostly bone.

The anhedonia has left me unable to enjoy anything and has all but extinguished my desire to consume. The more weight I lose, the heavier my mental burden.

One eye. Squinting. Daylight.

"Noooo, I can't," I sigh. "Not today."

I groan. Roll over. Grab the bedsheet and pull it over my head, blocking out light and sound.

I sense he is lying beside me. The sheet rises slightly with each inhalation and falls with each sigh. Oh yes, he is there, all right.

"Stop looking at me."

Is he looking at me? I think he is. I can feel his eyes burning through the sheet, trying to get my attention.

He is patient and kind, I reflect. Always there for me in the depths of my mental anguish. Even sleeps with me, not every night, but when I drag myself from fitful slumber, he is beside me.

My disdain for the world extends to everyone and everything but him, in fact. He is the one I can count on. Even when I can't count on myself. I shouldn't hate him. But sometimes I do. When he demands of me. When he wants me, and when I have nothing to give.

I curl tighter. He sighs, and reaches out to touch me.

"Don't . . ." I moan. "Please, not now."

He pushes me gently. *Come on. I need you. We need each other.*

"Noooo . . . I want to sleep," I whisper as I pull away. "I don't want to be awake. I want to be dead."

Sometimes the depression and anxiety rule my life. I sleep for twenty hours at a time. I don't eat. I don't drink. I don't have the energy to live. I wake up only to desire more of sleep's respite from the world. Many days I don't leave my bed.

I inch back the bedsheet, exposing first my tangled hair. Then forehead. Then eyes, first closed, then opening slowly, with apprehension. My face. The air outside my sheet shelter feels fresh and cool.

I glance in his direction. He is indeed gazing at me. He catches my eye and looks back with big, soulful brown eyes: *Hello. I love you.*

"Hi, buddy," I half sob. "I'm scared. I don't think I can."

You can. I love you. You will.

Let's.

He rises to his feet and lowers his face to my level. We're eye to eye. I can't escape.

And then he kisses me over and over, long slurpy pink-tongued kisses on my cheeks, my eyes, my nose. Licking me to life.

I throw back the sheet and extend my weary bones until my feet touch the floor.

His tail wags furiously with anticipation. *You're getting up, you're getting up, up, up, up!*

"Yeah, buddy, you win." I smile. "Just let me get dressed. Go get your leash and we'll go for a walk."

Catherine Kenwell is a Barrie, Ontario, author and mediator who sustained a mild traumatic brain injury in 2011. Prior to her accident, she enjoyed a thirty-year career in corporate communications. Post-injury, she lost her job, joined the circus, became a qualified mediator, and studied post-concussion brain rehabilitation. And yes, her dog saved her life.

SEEING JERRY

Jodie Toresdahl

A FAMILY OF RHINOS TAKES my attention away from my daughter. The parents are coaxing the two young ones to move along toward the next treat station. They have to manoeuvre past several princesses, a clunky Thomas the Tank Engine, and our very own two-year-old little Statue of Liberty to reach the prized bowl of Twix bars. The plaza at the Lincoln Center offers only five candy stations, but the costume watching makes it worth spending Halloween morning in the company of hundreds of other New York families.

After filling Norah's jack-o-lantern with Snickers and Skittles and suckers, we find a splash of sunlight between the shadows of the Metropolitan Opera House and the Library of Performing Arts to take a break and let Norah enjoy some of her spoils. She sits content with her lollipop dripping down to her sea-green Lady Liberty robe. I think it is the sticky red candy and parade of costume-clad children that are holding her attention while I chat with friends, but after a while she seems unusually calm despite the abundance of sugar and live characters.

I follow her gaze through the crowd to the benches across the walkway toward Juilliard's grass lawn. I see a family of mice, more princesses, and a proportional amount of tired parents—but nothing out of the ordinary for Halloween, so I turn back to my conversation. After several more minutes, I feel a tug on my arm. Norah looks up at me and simply smiles before walking toward the benches. I follow a few steps behind to see where her curious heart will lead.

As she approaches the bench, I see him. He has deep wrinkles on his face, and his lonely eyes cast downward, his back curling along with them. He sits alone in the midst of adults holding hands and children laughing, enjoying being together. The long black braids in his hair tell me the Native American coat he wears is not donned only one day a year—but rather with pride whenever it is cold enough to wrap around his shoulders.

Norah places her small hands on the bench next to him, and with incredible toddler strength, she vaults her way into the empty space beside him. She smiles and asks him his name. He mumbles something neither of us can understand. But as he mumbles, those deep wrinkles I think are set in a frown creak their way to a slight smile. His eyes still hold that loneliness, but they smile, too. Wisdom beyond her years tells Norah not to press him on his name like she typically does if she doesn't hear the answer she wants. As I sit in the spot next to her, she places her hand on his knee and says, "This is my new friend, Mom." Then, as if to explain why, she leans in to me and whispers, "He's an old man," and nods knowingly.

When she nods like that, I see my mom in my daughter. I think she is really trying to say, *I see Jerry in him.*

My mom is always noticing people like this man—people who seem to just need someone to acknowledge them. I remember one Christmas Eve when she came home an hour later than we were expecting her from work. She walked in the door, smiled, and told us about the young man at the store who was flustered because the person who was supposed to give him a ride to his friend's house for dinner never showed up. My mom watched him grow more anxious as he called everyone he knew and no one answered. So she told him to wait until the store closed at six, and she shuttled him where he needed to go, offering him a warm car and friendly, encouraging conversation to boot. It might seem careless to allow a stranger into your car and then let him tell you where to drive, but because my mom cared so much for people, she would do it anyway. "I could see Jerry in him" was always her reasoning, and we could never argue with that.

Jerry was my uncle—my mom's younger brother. I often wonder what he would have been like if the schizophrenia hadn't held him captive his entire adult life. That disease made his journey much more difficult than it needed to be. But our family's love was stronger than his disease. My grandparents and my mom, along with her siblings, fought for him louder than the voices did. He always had a seat at the table for after-Christmas games of Michigan rummy or left center right—even when he chose to spend many of those evenings smoking a pack of cigarettes in my grandparents' garage. When he was done and came huffing in the door, there would always be loud calls of, "Jerry! Come join us!" He never lasted more than a few hands before getting frustrated, but he wanted to be a part of the fun. You could tell by the twinkle in his eye when he smiled after winning a hand that he craved the company more than the silent garage. And while I will always wonder who he could have been, I will cherish who he was.

He was thoughtful when his disease allowed him to be selfless—like the Christmas shortly after Brett and I were married. Crumpled wrapping paper was piled in the middle of my grandparents' living room, and everyone was oohing and ahhing over their new gifts. Jerry got up slowly and reached his shaky hand into his pocket, coming out with a wad of five-dollar bills. He carefully made his way around the room, saying "Merry Christmas" as he handed one bill to each of us. He had exactly the right amount for each of his siblings, nieces, and nephew. That is the only gift I remember from that Christmas.

He was kind when he wasn't battling his demons—like the time a few years ago when my grandparents brought him to my parents' house so he could meet our daughter, his first great-niece. After a meal full of loud laughter and storytelling, all of the adults were in the kitchen cleaning up. I heard Norah's giggle over the clink of dishes in the sink and looked back to the dining room to find my six-month-old daughter in a deep, babbling conversation with her great-uncle Jerry. The kitchen grew quiet as we all watched the incredible connection forming between these two people who couldn't quite communicate to the rest of us the way they wanted to but found ease with each other.

I had these opportunities to see Jerry for who he was behind the dark schizophrenic cloud because he had a family who loved him fiercely and never gave up on him. My uncle died almost two years ago, but my mom hasn't stopped looking out for her younger brother. She has a heart that finds people who don't have the gift of a family who loves them fiercely like his did. She looks for the Jerry within the crowds and then takes action. Sometimes my dad is recruited in her efforts—like the time she had him come to the store, pick up a confused young man who needed a ride to the bus station, and buy his ticket to get back to his own big sister about an hour away. She got his sister's phone number, and once they connected, the woman offered to reimburse my mom for her kindness. My mom declined, saying she had a brother who would need someone to step in to help him sometimes, too.

There is a lot of discernment that goes into knowing who to help and how to help them. I'm glad my mom's Jerry-sense seems to have rubbed off on my daughter. I hope I can learn from both of them.

The old man's smile is still on his face when Norah turns back toward him after her knowing nod toward me. That nod that says, *I see Jerry in him, Mom. He needs us to be his family right now.* My instinct is to get up and walk through the crowd back toward the comfortable circle of friends who are waiting for us. But Norah sits firmly, and the man seems to sit a bit taller with my daughter beside him. My two-year-old daughter sees Jerry in this man, and I am sure my mom would have seen him, too. Norah needs me to sit with her so we can be his family for a moment. So we stay. We sit on the bench, an awkward family of three, watching costumes in silence, and no one is alone.

Jodie Toresdahl is a Montana girl at heart, living her dream life in New York City with her husband and daughter, who both love adventure as much as she does. She writes about raising a child in New York, learning from the thousands of encounters with people she meets there, and growing through the discomfort of transition at bigskytobigapple.com.

CANDLE IN THE WIND

Jorden Mathias

WHILE ON HER DEATH BED, frail and beautiful, my mom tells me to watch for the butterflies. "I will be with you when you see them," she says with what voice she has left. "They will protect you."

Not long after she takes her last breath, I vow not only to remember her spirit every time I see a butterfly but also to get clean and sober . . . finally. I'm a self-proclaimed junkie—an addict of the grievous variety. And recovery isn't going to be easy.

Working with my brother shortly after my mom's death is a gift, as my addiction has cost me many jobs. But I am having a bad day—my withdrawals are agonizing. I'm feeling nauseous and weak, and I really just want a drink or a drug to ease the pain I am experiencing. I have a moment of self-pity as I hammer some deck boards together. *I wish my mom was still here. I miss her so much.* Then suddenly, my brother yells over to me, "There's a butterfly near your head." I look up. There she is, beautiful and so . . . there! I put my hand up to see if I can touch her, and she lands on it. Soft green, yellow, and brown wings flutter slowly while her legs grasp onto my palm. My brother snaps a picture.

Suddenly my withdrawal symptoms slip away. I am at peace for a moment; it's as if my mom is holding my hand.

That night, still in awe of what I experienced with the soft green butterfly, I look for documentaries about butterflies and find one with a butterfly on the cover. The film isn't about butterflies per se, but rather about grief and loss—I am drawn to it immediately. It's about a camp for grieving children—heartbreaking—and how they perform certain ceremonies to help them heal from the painful loss they experienced. One of the rituals is to write their lost parent a letter and to release it into a fountain to symbolize letting them go in a peaceful way.

I call my twelve-step sponsor as soon as the documentary is finished. "I have an idea," I say to him. He's always on board with helping me. He and his girlfriend humour me and meet me at the waterfront in my hometown the next day.

When we all arrive at the shore of a nearby lake, I am excited to pull out some plates, candles, paper, and pens from a bag. "Okay, both of you need to write down a fear that you want to get rid of," I say. "Then we are going to light them on fire and send the candles out into the bay to truly release them."

So far they seem to be happy with the idea, but my sponsor notices something that will make this event difficult. "Couldn't you find any candles that were shorter?" he chuckles. "Those won't stand up on the plate, Jorden. They are too tall."

I didn't think about that, but they were the only candles I could find. "We will have to try our best, I suppose," I reply, determined to perform the ritual.

It's a chilly Halloween night. Our fingers, cold from the soft wind blowing from the water, write out the fears we want to release, and I also write a letter to my mom. I want to say goodbye and feel at peace. The pain of losing her is still so great, and I am hopeful that this ceremony will bring me some serenity.

"Okay, I will go first," says my sponsor. He lights his fear successfully and burns it away. But as soon as he pushes the candle out into the water, it tips over and goes out.

Then my sponsor's girlfriend gives it a try—same result, fear turned to ash, a soggy candle, and a plate bobbing in the waves.

"Okay, let's give this one more kick at the can," I say, not too confident that my candle will be anything but also scientifically incapable of standing long enough to make it a foot from the shore. But then something happens; it stays lit and standing for five whole feet. The chilly waves try to bring it back to shore, but then it gets taken out farther and farther. I look at my sponsor and his girlfriend. We are all speechless as we sit on the sand and watch as it travels out far past our reach. The full moon shines onto the water and makes the reflection of the candlelight on the waves look like a trail of tears streaming from the plate as it travels out even farther into the bay.

A boat passes by. *This will be the end of it, I'm sure*, I think. But as the waves get bigger, the plate gracefully rides them and doesn't let the candle fall. The three of us watch in awe and silence. Two and a half hours later, the candle is still burning. As we leave the waterfront, we pass a mom and a son sitting near the water—I am confident it is not a coincidence. As we make our way back to the car, we take one last look from the hill and my sponsor says to me, "I think your mom's telling you that she will be with you forever." *No drink or drug could possibly give me this high*, I think as we warm up in the car and reflect on the experience we just shared.

The next morning a friend is taking me to renew my licence, and as we pull up to a red light, a Monarch butterfly lands on the windshield directly in front of my eyes. It doesn't mean much to my friend, but it means everything to me. *Hi, Mom,* I think to myself with a smile on my face. *Thank you for always being with me. I hope you liked your candle.*

Approximately nine months go by, and on my one-year sobriety anniversary, my sponsor gives me a card and the inscription says, A CANDLE IN THE WIND, LIKE NO OTHER.

Jorden Mathias is a dad to three beautiful children and is also a new grandpa. He has been in recovery from drug and alcohol addiction for three years. He has his own general contracting company and enjoys baseball, volleyball, and helping other addicts achieve recovery by volunteering at a local detox centre. He also is a musician and enjoys writing his own songs. He's a family guy all around.

MARATHON

Terri Lynn Futcher

WE WAKE UP EARLY AND prepare our bodies to run our first marathon together as a young and newly married couple.

"Hope it was worth the effort," I say to Chris through nervous glances as we put on our carefully prepared race-day outfits.

We are just two numbers in the chaos of thirty thousand. We have trained for this day for months, completing run after gruelling training run together. My view is his backside as he pulls me along to finish each run in preparation for the big day. I wouldn't have started without him, and I most certainly wouldn't finish.

Physical pain is something he can block out or duel with, winning every time. For me, it is sheer misery, my body begging me to stop every single day. But as a newlywed trying to impress her husband, I let him pull me along, right up to today as we join the flood of runners in downtown Tokyo, Japan, and start the race together.

As we join the masses at the start line and are on display to the thousands of cheering spectators, our glances have changed from uncertain to confident. Yes, the seemingly endless preparation was worth it.

We feel strong. We feel healthy. We feel prepared. As we log each of the forty-two kilometres, we are bound by the time we'd spent together preparing. We are proud of each other. We enjoy the sideline swarms of cheers, assuming the Japanese drums and chants are to congratulate and encourage us. As we approach the last few kilometres, that pain thing starts to overtake my struggling legs and failing mind. Just slow down. Take it easy. Maybe even stop. But every time, I look up and see his strong legs and consistent pace. He looks back at me after every few strides, willing me to keep up, keep going, press forward.

"Come on," he says over his shoulder. "We can see the finish line. If we can get there in fifty-four seconds, we will reach our goal."

So I pick it up, wanting to make him proud more than wanting to reach our goal. In fifty-three seconds, we cross the line, just one second faster than our goal. Runners continue to swarm past the finish, some rejoicing, some vomiting, but all in victory. He is the reason I could do it. He is the reason I even wanted to do it.

I push out our first adorably cute baby about a year later. A beautiful mix of Hawaiian, Chinese, and Caucasian makes our children look less like mine and much more like his. The dark hair, the brown eyes, and the rich complexions raise questions as I tote them around town.

"Well, they sure don't look like you, do they?" I hear a lady at the grocery store say.

I respond with pride, "Their dad is Hawaiian."

I want him to have the credit. He busies himself with starting and growing a very successful media company. We are well taken care of. We spoil the kids with little and big luxuries and start putting away for the future. Our ducks are, as they say, in a row. The only sign is stress. Having his own business leads to struggles and challenges we don't know how to handle.

Marriage becomes increasingly challenging as kids take over time and attention. And that is what leads to the day.

It is a day that starts like any other. Feed the kids. Change the baby's diaper. Do the dishes. Feed the dog. It progresses quickly to what is frighteningly and seemingly unreal. He becomes increasingly confused—off—slipping into what appears to be a different world. Looking into his eyes is like looking into the eyes of someone on a TV screen—you can see him but he can't see you back. He's somewhere else. He starts seeing things that are somewhere else, too. The kids cling. The baby coos. He is gentle but increasingly overcome by stress and anxiety, as he knows he is unable to be reached. It continues to progress quickly. Before I know who is there or what is happening, I am nursing my baby on the top bunk of my kids' bed as I send my son to the backyard and let my older daughter in the closed room with me. I draw the curtain, but it doesn't block out the sound of the sirens and the paramedics physically removing him from our idyllic home on the tree-lined street we'd ridden our bikes down so often.

The next couple of days are as horrific for him as they are for me. As he is strapped down, hands and feet, in a small locked room guarded by a stranger, I am home in bed, unable to lift the covers. My baby lies beside me, trying to nurse out milk that just isn't being produced. As my husband is in the intensive care psych ward, I am begged to just drink something. It's surprising, sometimes, how you can go from relying on someone to propel you forward to wondering if he'll be able to pull himself up again. After a few days of "other world" experiences, his mind settles into our realm once again, and the physicians let him come home with no diagnosis. "Lack of sleep," the doctor says.

Life changes. My husband struggles with trying to feel again, trying to relate, and trying to be understood. I struggle with getting to know the person he is now, trying to relate again, and trying to understand. I can no longer let him pull me. I have to find the victories myself and learn how to get to them on my own. I have to be the one who shows up each day, not knowing if he will be able to or not. Some days he can't get out of bed before noon. Others he can conquer getting up by two p.m. Regular social gatherings become too much for him, and everyday-life stresses are out of the question.

I guess some would say I am pulling him this time. Instead of the goal of a respectable marathon finish time, I have my sights set on a future of function for us and our growing children. I pick up the slack. I make excuses for him. I become the family spokesperson and smile big enough for both of us so that others will think we are okay. I'd like to think that he knows this is the time he can let me pull him.

Time really does produce change. Sometimes it brings the kind of change we hope for, and other times it brings the change we dread. This time, it has gifted us with healing. But maybe that isn't true. Time didn't do it. He did. As I am smiling to the world, he is behind the scenes, feeling the pain that comes with mental illness, wrapped up in the confusion of what happened, what is, and what will be. He keeps going, even though this time it is he who is hurting, he whose mind is telling him to stop. Today, he starts to run again after almost a decade of stillness. As his pace increases, his mind seems to gain clarity. As his stride finds its rhythm again, his person—his true inner person—finds its cadence. Once again, I'm watching him take the lead, pull me along, overcome the pain. Tomorrow might be different. I might find myself looking over my shoulder at him, silently willing him to come. He might look ahead, not sure if it's worth the effort.

But today, right now, he has his head forward and his mind clear. Today, we feel strong, healthy, and prepared again. I am confident that we will reach our goals together once more. I don't know who will pull whom and what the various finish lines will look like. But I know, from experience, that it's okay for the run to turn out a little differently than we thought it would. Things will change. We will learn. We will even take turns pulling each other along. But we will continue forward.

Terri Lynn Futcher enjoys spending time with her kids on their small hobby farm, running, and taking photos for Kaspi Creative, the stock-photography business started by and run by her husband. Chris can now far outrun her, although she tries to keep up. She is thankful they are both running in the right direction. Check out their website at kaspi.ca.

LOVE ME

Heather Down

MY ABILITY TO SWIM IS only slightly surpassed by my ability to text, which is marginally better than my ability to twitter on the tweeting machine—and, unfortunately, I perform those tasks so well, it qualifies me to run for leader of the free world. When it comes to texting, half of the time my fingers hit the wrong buttons, half of the time the autocorrect has a different agenda, and the other half of the time I have the keyboard set to French. Is that too many halves? Oh well, you get my drift.

I accompany some folks who are part of a band to a small town where they are playing in a theatre. During the afternoon sound check, I explore the metropolis of Meaford, population 10,991 and a half (Mrs. Jones is expecting baby number three). I find myself very hungry, standing in front of the local coffee shop at exactly 3:02 p.m., face streaming with tears, because apparently in Meaford, coffee shops close at three p.m. What? Does no one drink coffee past three o'clock in rural parts of Canada?

I have no data on my phone to google any alternatives, so in typical Heather fashion, I text my friend Natalie for advice:

Me: Did u knew the coffae ship in Meaford class at 3? What kand if town is tis???

Nat: Huh? Lol.

Me: Thay id doing soins check for tonught si I an winder-ing aimlessly.

Nat: You need to get your blood sugars up before you text lol!

Me: OMH, Yeis.

Nat: Do you need an ambulance girl?

Me: Haha. I just fawnd anuther café. Catering plase. It us culled Kitchen.

Nat: Simple enough. Are they going to feed you so that you can text in English?

Me: Hahah . . . I hop sow lol.

Later that week my friend Tammy and I pop into Natalie's for a couple of minutes. Upon leaving, we see a loose dog wandering the streets. The sweet little dog appears to be confused, and we try to corral her in hopes of keeping her safe. I text Natalie: We need u. We need a leash. Natalie assumes I am up to my hypoglycemic texting tricks again.

Nat: Lol! Oh Heather. Get some sugar in your body!

Me: Nope lol.

This obviously isn't going to plan. Trying to clarify the confusing situation, I try again.

Me: Dooug.

Nat: Yes. Lol! I'm Peron laughing.

Peron laughing? Who's hypoglycemic now, Natalie?

Me: Huh?

Nat: Oooops! Peeing.

I still don't have a leash. Finally, Natalie hangs her head out the window, and we clear up my texting fiasco. Natalie and her son, Adam, come outside with a leash. She kindly takes the dog to the local vet, and luckily thirteen-year-old Bebe is micro-chipped and is returned to her rightful owner.

As mentioned, my swimming skills are probably even worse. However, with a torn anterior cruciate ligament and twenty-five percent of my meniscus gone in my right knee (knowledge courtesy of a painful MRI—the MRI itself didn't hurt; however, a half hour of listening to Sarah McLachlan's *Mirrorball* piped into my brain through the earphones was akin to torture), I need some type of physical activity. Running was my saviour. It was the only way I could get the anxiety out. I would start a run agitated, unfocused, and unquieted, only to feel the emotion depleting little by little with every footfall.

I saw a T-shirt once that read RUNNING—CHEAPER THAN THERAPY. Whoever came up with that slogan never paid full price for a pair of high-end running shoes.

So in its stead, my friend Lyndsay and I plan on going swimming together. Now, there is something you should know: Lyndsay and I have the combined organizational skills of a six-month-old. In fact, I identify her car not by the license plate but by looking in the back seat. If it looks like the residence of three families, complete with four kids and a dog, I know I have the right vehicle. Even the most populous back alleys of Mumbai can't rival the interior of her car—a scene straight out of *Slumdog Millionaire*. I remember looking in once to see one high-heeled shoe, countless paper coffee cups, a half-eaten bagel, a macramé project, and possibly a dead body (I can't be sure).

Given this information, it is no surprise how the following text thread starts:

Lyndsay: How are you feeling about swimming? Still able to? I have to find my stuff.

Me: I have to find my stuff, too.

No shocker here. It's only the morning of the planned event and neither of us has bothered to locate any of our swimming gear.

Lyndsay: Okay. Great.

Me: I have found everything except swimsuit and lock.

Which is only half true. I had found two locks, both locked permanently to my swim bag because I can't remember the combinations.

Lyndsay: Okay . . . I need to find my goggles and lock.

(two minutes later)

Me: Found suit.

Lyndsay: Found lock. Just need goggles. I'm very excited. I have to spend some time primping first.

Me: I found two pairs of goggles now.

(two-minute pause)

Lyndsay: I think we should swim more regularly to keep up on grooming habits and gentle reminders of what it feels like to squeeze yourself into sausage casing.

I am laughing pretty hard right now, but that isn't the punchline.

Lyndsay: My suit is so tight it's correcting my posture . . .

On the way to the pool, I go out to the dollar store to find a replacement lock. Knowing that this predicament occurs every time I stop swimming for over a week, I pick up one, no two— what the heck—four locks. They are only three dollars each. I guess the word "dollar" in dollar store is metaphorical.

I get home and put on my suit, but it seems to have altered. It has been over a year; what could possibly change? It appears that the elastic in the bit that is supposed to snuggly cover my bottom has given up, completely losing its will to live. There is a full inch of slack between the material and my backside, causing the suit to naturally ride up in a sort of permanent wedge-y position. It is incredibly uncomfortable and awkward for me, but not nearly as awkward as it will be for anyone who will have to witness the sight.

Upon arrival at the pool, Lyndsay and I chat about the beautiful day: "It is so nice out today. We could have swum in the lake," Lyndsay mentions.

"Yeah, that way we wouldn't have to ingest all that toxic chlorine. We could drink the oil from the boats and the refuse from the city's water treatment plant instead," I chirp cheerfully.

"Yeah, except here we are in a controlled environment so that when we start to drown, we are more likely to be rescued."

"True dat." And into the pool we go.

Although running is my preferred form of exercise, I tolerate swimming because it seems like it should be the quickest route to Michelle Obama arms. I love her shoulders. I would give anything to wear one of those tops with cut-out arms and look like her. I tried on one of those blouses once, and I looked less like Michelle Obama and more like Buddhist prayer flags flapping at Mount Everest Base Camp.

Slow and steady—the emphasis on slow (after all, it is called front *crawl*)—we traverse the pool, back and forth like pensioners walking laps around the perimeter of our long-term care facility in our zoom-a-frames. And it feels . . . good. Moving meditation. That is what I miss most about running: the space between the moments when you float, suspended. Now, here in the pool, there are no worries of miscommunication or bathing suits that have failed me or the craziness of the world. I allow my mind to be free, leaving my demons to sink and my optimism to float. I simply focus on one arm in front of the other. And since I am such a bad swimmer, I really MUST focus solely on this movement . . . or I will drown. Literally. I am serious. I swim like a rock. The stakes are kind of high: lift arm, *don't drown*, pull arm through water, *don't drown*, breathe, *don't drown*, repeat.

After the peaceful swim, we somehow find ourselves at Starbucks. How does that always happen? I enjoy chatting and catching up and think, *Why don't I make more time for these types of moments, moments of laughing and peace, moments for* ME?

Self-care and mental wellness are so important. It takes practice to schedule these ever-crucial activities into my life, simple joys that can keep me well. Instead, I often choose to drown in my daily challenges instead of being buoyed by everyday pleasures. I don't want to forget this realization, so I type a note to myself on my phone. Just like my texting ability, sometimes it takes several times to get it right:

Me: Live moi

Me: Loue maw

DARN IT!

Me: Love me!

It's a work in progress. But eventually, lap by lap, I get there in the end.

You can read all about Heather Down's incredible misadventures at themoosepyjamachronicles.blogspot.ca.

MORE THAN A DOUGHNUT

Karen Copeland

WE ARE STUCK IN AN airport because of bad weather. My children are restless. I am on my own with them, and after a hectic weekend full of visiting numerous relatives, we are all ready to be home.

And then it happens. Despite all his best efforts, my son begins to experience a significant challenge. On the surface it appears like a child having a temper tantrum. But if you have a child on the spectrum, or one who experiences a high level of anxiety, you will also know it is much more than that. I spring into survival mode—desperately trying to help him manage and cope. It's not easy in these moments because other eyes are upon you, and you wonder about the thoughts behind their stares. I know what I have to do. My approach is different than other parents' may be, but I know this will work best. We spend a great deal of time getting to a calm state, and when we finally arrive, he asks for a doughnut from the airport coffee shop.

The three of us walk over to the kiosk, and I order the doughnuts. Sitting down on a bench, I feel exhausted but glad we have averted something much bigger until I hear my son say, "This isn't the one I asked for." And I know the risk of escalation is now upon us once again. Looking up, I see the line has grown to more than twenty people.

I gather up the courage to approach a woman near the front of the line. I venture, "If I give you some money, could you buy me a chocolate-glazed doughnut?"

"You can go ahead of me in the line," the stranger offers.

"Thank you, but no. Would it be possible for you to purchase the doughnut and bring it over to us?" I say, gesturing toward the row of seats where my family temporarily resides.

"Okay," she smiles.

She buys the doughnut and brings it over to us. I almost cry because she does so without any looks of judgment.

I say, "I can't thank you enough. How things appear on the surface aren't always exactly what's going on, and you have no idea how much you've helped us today."

It would have been easy for her to have looked at me like I was the mother giving in to her misbehaving child. She could have refused to purchase the doughnut and told me to go to the end of the line. She could have allowed that look to come across her eyes that told me she disagreed, but she didn't. And because she didn't, she threw us a life preserver that assisted us to make it through the rest of our day.

Months later, I am in an airport again, waiting for my flight. There is a mom standing in line at the coffee kiosk, and her children are running around, playing. Mom is calling quite loudly for the kids to come stand beside her to no avail. Two ladies sitting behind me begin to comment and say, "Well, guess what she's in for if she can't even get her kids to listen to her now. Guess what will happen when they are teenagers."

And I think of the woman who helped us. It might have seemed like such a small thing to do for a family, but it wasn't—it was such a big help.

I silently thank her again, grateful it was she who was in the airport that day.

Karen Copeland has two children, one of whom experiences mental health and other challenges. Karen started writing about her parenting experiences in 2014 in efforts to generate more understanding about the difficulties that exist in obtaining the care her family needs and deserves. You can follow her blog at championsforcommunitywellness.com.

PRAISE

Reema Sukumaran

"MAX, ZACK, HURRY UP. I don't want to be late. Your dad, Tyler, and Jordan are on the praise team this week," I yell up the stairs. I am trying desperately to get six sons between the ages of thirteen and twenty-one to the church on time—*literally*.

We pile into two cars, my husband, Sanj, driving the car and Max driving the SUV. Sanj helps people hear in two entirely different ways—during the week he is an audiologist, and on the weekend he is a part of creating beautiful music at our church.

I scurry into my usual pew. I like to sit in the third row back on the left. The music begins, and my heart swells with pride. I look up at Sanj, Tyler, and Jordan as they share their talents, leading the congregation in song. It is a good moment, a very good moment.

Not like many of the moments of my childhood—abusive father, battered mother, raped by a pastor. I have all the cliché characters in my personal trauma story. I would experience new disruptions and carefully and quietly fold them into neat little squares that I meticulously stacked on top of previous squares of repressed emotions deep within my psyche.

I appreciate my current life. A lot. I appreciate it because normal is relative. My life is sometimes full and chaotic—some would say crazy, even. But it isn't ugly. Not like it used to be.

I thought I had dealt with the fallout of my past, the hand I was dealt. My clever mind tried to deceive me into believing this to be truth, as it convinced me nothing sinister was hiding within the secret folds of its grey matter. However, my body knew better.

"Mom, are you okay?" my sons and husband would sometimes ask.

But I was anything but.

It crept up, insipid and unchecked. Surprising me because the changes weren't noticed until they were no longer just changes; they were *transformations*.

Occasional panic attacks spread unchecked, growing into debilitating fear. Post-traumatic stress reared its sinister head, rendering me incapable of doing even the simplest of things. I couldn't be left alone. My friends had to babysit me during the day until my boys could pick me up and take me home. Then Sanj would come home from work and take over.

Sleep. Exist. Can't be left alone. Repeat.

Back in the church, the praise team starts a new song. It triggers a Herculean memory dating back to the previous January:

"Hey, Reema, would you like to come with us to shop for Alexx's prom dress?" my friend Penny asked. Penny's daughter and my son, Tyler, were dates for the upcoming prom.

"Of course," I answered.

Tyler drove, and Alexx sat in the front while Penny and I settled into the back.

But something started to happen. First I simply felt off, but it escalated to more, way more.

"Are you okay?" Penny asked.

I didn't answer. I was unable to. My thoughts and feelings seemed unreal, as if they belonged to someone else. I was slipping from myself and couldn't stop it. I was losing "me."

"Pull over," Penny instructed Tyler. "There is a gas station ahead." She told Alexx to call 9-1-1.

I became violent, seizing uncontrollably.

"Ouch," Penny screamed as my out-of-control flailing limbs caught her nose.

"Mom, Mom . . ." Tyler tried to reach me, the me that was escaping wildly, depersonalizing.

Sirens. Paramedics. Restraints. Handcuffs.

"Please don't be so rough with her," Tyler pleaded. "She . . . she's my mother."

He climbed into the ambulance with me, not leaving my side.

Tests. Follow-ups. Medical visits. Inconclusive.

Back at home, I continued to be supervised at all times. Exhausted and petrified, I raced from the shower for fear someone was behind me even though, logically, I knew that wasn't possible.

Depression. Fear. Frustrations. Sadness.

My mind jolts back to the present moment in church as a new song begins. It triggers me in every way possible.

Notes. Sound. Music. Message.

Everyone is on their feet. I attempt to rise but can't. I am cemented to the pew. A wave of emotion ruptures from the depths of my buried trauma, washing over and consuming me, pinning me down, paralyzing me. My shoulders shake visibly. I cry so deeply, it is silent—silent tears always roar the loudest.

Catharsis. Release. Unfolding.

But in that moment I am lonely. Lonely, swimming in my pool of pain. Lonelier than I have ever been in my entire life. But that only lasts for a split second.

Then I feel an arm circle my shoulder. I manage to look at the person beside me. Sally, a woman I barely know, has spotted me. She holds me, without judgment, without questions, without expectation. I am not alone. Soon other women join us, and we huddle in a loving embrace.

I am here. I am loved. I am getting better.

Praise.

Reema Sukumaran is a wife to an amazing husband, and together they are journeying in this life with six wonderful sons. Reema is a blogger, a speaker, and a survivor of clergy sexual abuse. She has used her pain to help others through advocating and educating. She suffers from mental illness, but it does not define her. To learn about Reema and her speaking availability, please visit reematalks.com.

IN THE DARK OF NIGHT

Courtney Taylor

"I JUST WANT TO KILL MYSELF," he wails through the phone. It's late. Or is it early? It's that time when night is flirting with early morning; it's midnight dark out, yet I can hear the birds have already begun their chorus. I hear them outside my window, and I hear them on his end of the phone, singing their premature song to him while he despairs.

It's near three a.m. on a Sunday, a year and a half since my last bout of depression.

I can't say if that time in October 2016 was the worst of all my worst times; I find it hard to recall the pain of the episodes previous. When stuck in the thick muck of a dark depression, it's hard to imagine one will ever forget the palpable clarity of the pain, but it does seem to recede into the past over time. I do know, however, that during that despondent period of time almost two years ago, the most severe moment of a life permeated with anxiety and depression took place.

In the midst of wrestling with the thoughts the illness was orchestrating in my mind, suicide appeared to me as a viable option for the very first time. The mere suggestion of its availability, and the quick question of *how?* that followed, filled me with more anguish and fear than I'd ever felt before.

In a crumpled heap on my floor, I sobbed in what became even physical agony, my wails of distress echoing through the quiet emptiness of my home, frightening my dog.

Though moving from my position on the carpet to locate my phone felt like my Everest, I did eventually reach out to a friend for help, and approximately two weeks later I was starting to see the light again.

Because of this experience, I know the depths of despair one can feel; I understand why people choose suicide. I know that kind of pain. I've met it head on, I've tried to run from it, and I've been knocked down by it. I've been there.

And he knew that.

So it's near three a.m. on a Sunday, 2:44 a.m. to be exact. I'm fast asleep. I hear my phone, but I'm not sure if I'm dreaming. By the time I'm conscious enough, it stops ringing. I must have immediately fallen back to sleep.

3:02 a.m. My phone rings again. I rouse enough to identify who's calling, and I pick up.

"Hello?" I say, gently. After a beat, he says hi, and then silence. I speak his name, as a question, really. Only his name, only one syllable, heavy with questions. The line goes dead.

Confused, my mind now clearing from middle-of-the-night fog, I realize I have a voice mail. It's him. His voice is calm, casual. Measured. He apologizes for bothering me, acknowledges that I'm probably asleep, and asks me to call if I get his message.

3:06 a.m. I call him back. He picks up, and I say his name, again as a question, and then I hold my breath.

I can barely decipher the words through his strained, sob-filled voice, but I do.

"I just want to kill myself," he wails. I can hear the pain in his words, sharp like the blade of a knife. Just muttering the words aloud cuts him inside, I can tell. His mind is full of demons, his heart is holding onto every memory he's made as a paramedic. He's been off work for almost three months, hoping time and space might act as a healing balm on his soul. He's been trying, but he's one man attempting to row a huge, heavy boat upstream, and he can't do it by himself. I've been trying to tell him this, but his shame and his stigma keep him adrift alone on this dark sea, and tonight a storm has come in. He's drowning.

"Where are you?" I ask him, keeping my tone calm, my voice steady. *No sudden movements*, I tell myself. *Keep the panic out of your voice.*

He's at home. He's been drinking.

We've only met once, for dinner, at a restaurant right around the corner from his condo. We both had pasta, and we shared an apple-rhubarb crumble for dessert. He had a beer. I had a cider. He was able to walk home from the restaurant; that's how close he lives. There are a few condos there, but I don't know which one is his. I don't know his address.

I ask him for it, my voice serene, making sure I don't sound like I'm begging. He's not really hearing me. He just keeps telling me he's sorry. Sorry for bothering me, sorry for everything.

"Go back to sleep. I'm sorry I woke you," he says between cries.

"Naw, I'm good. No worries. I'm actually kind of hungry. Maybe I'll have an early breakfast . . ." I try to play it down, try to reassure him he has no need to be sorry.

I ask him if he's made a plan. He has.

I ask him if he's prepared anything to act out his plan. He has. He's tied a cable to the railing of his tenth-floor balcony.

I have to get help. I have to get help.

He doesn't want to die. He wouldn't have called me if he did. He called me for help. He's crying out, literally, for help. I have to get help.

Holding the phone up to my ear, I'm suddenly frighteningly aware of the fact that I have no other means to call for help. I haven't had a land line in years. I'll have to let him go to make the 9-1-1 call. My mind races, frantically searching for solutions to avoid disconnecting from him.

I come up with none.

"Do you want me to come?" I ask, without any intention of actually going.

His voice shakes through his tears and he replies, "Only if you want to."

"Why don't I come?" I say. Then, "Listen, I just have to do a couple of things to get ready to come there, okay? Just give me like five minutes and I'll call you right back. Stay where you are, okay? Just stay there. I'm going to call you back in less than five minutes, okay?" I keep repeating myself at least four times, and when I'm confident in his compliance, I hang up and quickly dial 9-1-1.

It rings. And rings. Then, "Thank you for calling Emergency Services. Please hold and your call will be answered in priority sequence."

"Dammit!" I say aloud.

I don't have time to sit on hold. I don't even have the time to give them all the details they need. All he needs is seconds to make that decision, to stand up, to take the next step. I have to get him back on the phone. I have to keep him here.

3:25 a.m. I call my neighbour, and she answers on the fourth ring. She knows it's me. She assumes I'm the one in need, that I'm having a panic attack, and that I need help, comfort, care. I quickly tell her I need to use her phone, and why, then proceed to run down the sidewalk in my Blue Jays nightshirt, my housecoat flung over my shoulder, my phone already redialling his number.

I enter a home I've entered hundreds of times before, and I hand her a piece of paper on which I've scribbled his address (which he did finally provide) and his name. I mute my phone to tell her I need her to talk to the dispatcher since I've got to stay on the phone with him, and I don't want him to know they're on their way, or he may panic and I might lose him.

Everything seems to slow down as my neighbour relays information to the dispatcher. "Yes, he's been drinking . . . No, no drugs . . . Yes, he's alone . . . No, no weapons, I don't think."

"He's a paramedic with the region," I want them to know. "He'll be worried about who shows up at his door."

None of his co-workers know what he's been going through. Neither do his friends or his family. His parents don't even know that for weeks he's been off work. For a quick second, I allow myself to wonder what might have happened if I didn't know, if he wasn't able to call me. I shake the thought away, clearing it like an Etch A Sketch, and ask him if he's still on his balcony.

"Why don't you go inside?" I encourage.

He refuses. He wants the fresh air. I get it. I've hungered for that same air many times, standing outside in the dead of night, gulping down massive breaths of air as if I were suffocating. And in a way, I was. Sometimes in the midst of winter, when panic wouldn't allow me time to put on boots and a parka, I'd open a window and press my face against its companion screen, cold winds slapping my skin, the synthetic smell of the wire mesh bringing to mind the last time I kissed its surface. The fresh air helped slow my breathing. Drawing it in, exhaling it back out, my breath hovering mid-air, carrying the cloud of anxiety away.

Knowing he's still on his balcony makes me nervous, but I don't let it show. I keep him engaged, I try to keep our conversation flowing. I try to reassure him, soothe him, calm him. His cries have quieted down a bit; he's not as hysterical as he was before. But he's still speaking of his desire to cease to exist, his desire to feel nothing.

He asks me, "What's the point?" I run an imaginary highlighter through my memory, trying to retrieve the notes I've been taught during training for just this circumstance. I don't remember how I answer, or the specific words I say. My tongue feels thick in my mouth, and my throat is dry. Adrenaline is doing somersaults in my abdomen. I just know I told him it was possible to get better, that he could get through this, to just hang on. Hang on. Hang on.

Minutes feel like hours, heavy with the threat of death. He could drop the phone at any moment, without warning, because the warning has already been raised. I know the stakes. I know something as simple as saying the wrong word could mean the difference between his life and his death. So I try to keep my mind clear, my voice kind and understanding, and my heart full of hope.

My neighbour stands in the dimly lit living room, listening to me talk to him, parroting my words to the call taker. Our conversations are separate, yet intertwined, separate threads that make up one rope. She mouths, "The police have arrived at the building." I'm thankful he has not spotted them from his tenth-floor perch. I know it's only a matter of moments now and he'll be safe. Physically safe.

Then I hear them. Voices other than his or mine—the police. I hear him answer them, before he says to me, "You called the cops?" and then, "I'm going to hang up now."

I think I mutter, "Okay," and then he's gone. But he's alive. I exhale and sit back in my neighbour's chair. The bits of breath I've been holding release, and I allow myself to relax. I think I whisper, "Oh thank God," or something similar, as my eyes sting with the threat of tears.

My neighbour looks at me, then at her watch, smiles with relief, and says, "Cup of tea?"

"Yes," I say. As I listen to her fill the kettle in the next room, my mind wanders back to that day in October almost two years ago when I had a day not so different from the one my paramedic friend has just endured. I was rescued, too. Not from what you might call immediate danger, not from a plan I had set into motion, but from the same kind of pain. From the same feelings of hopelessness, the same desire to feel anything but the nothing I was feeling. I was served tea that day, too, when I was on the other end of the call for help.

I'm brought back to the present moment when my cellphone rings. It's a sergeant with the region, still at the scene, wanting me to know that my friend is on his way to the hospital. He tells me that all the information I had provided was accurate, and then he says four words I'll never forget: *You saved his life.*

Depression is torture, and every day I hope and pray it will never return and invade my brain. It is an army of darkness, a force that can destroy, turn technicolour to black and white. The moments I have faced in the harsh, oppressive hold of mental illness have been the worst of my life. But in this moment, I realize that the pain I have withstood when held in its maddening grip has been transformed into a weapon I can yield to save others from its suffocation.

I am struck with the ironic knowledge that had I never experienced that deep black void for myself, I may not have been able to help another survive theirs. It turns out that my best moments have grown from the roots of my worst, like a spring flower that emerges from what appears to be a dead and dark frozen earth. The ability to help others as I have been helped is certainly an unexpected gift for which I could not be more grateful.

Upon his release from the hospital just over a day later, my friend reaches out to tell me he is more motivated than ever to get better. I listen as he shares his plan to confide in his family later that evening, and I cannot ignore the bittersweet beauty hidden in the silent, agonizing corners of my depression and anxiety, the beauty that lives in knowing no greater triumph than the triumph that is born out of tragedy. Even when born in the dark of night.

Courtney Taylor lives with generalized anxiety disorder and emetophobia and has experienced four severe depressive episodes. A former volunteer with Partners for Mental Health, she is the co-founder of March for Mental Health, Toronto. Trained in mental health first aid and safeTALK, as well as being a CMHA certified psychological health and safety advisor, she is currently assisting Ontario MP Charlie Angus with the development of Parliamentary Motion M-174 #NotOneMore, which calls on the Canadian government to implement a National Suicide Prevention Action Plan.

She works in legal publishing, where she assists her HR department in the execution of mental health and wellness workplace initiatives. She lives in Toronto with her dog.

BEING A PARENT IS SOBERING

Serge Gagné

I GET OUT OF THE shower after work to a pile of printed text messages from "the other woman" on the bed. I turn around to the sound of my wife telling me that "We are done"—cold, solemn, and heartbroken. The devastation in her eyes betrays her. I start to cry as I pack my bags. How did she find out? How did I become so selfish? My kids! How could I hurt my sweet children? How?

Growing up, I didn't have many positive role models in my life. My mom and dad were alcoholics and were often absent. I was lonely and felt like I didn't belong in this world. When I was twelve, I started sneaking cigarettes from my mom, and I began experimenting with drugs and alcohol. Suddenly, instantly, immediately, I could numb the pain, get out of my head, and time warp into the in-crowd. I figured I had found the solution to all my problems. This false sense of euphoria really worked . . . until it didn't.

One thing I knew for sure, however, was that I would never grow up to be like my parents. My resolve to not be like my parents became daily thoughts. Then I would feel guilty about feeling this way and would numb myself even more with substances that offered only temporary relief.

Now, I have lost my wife and no longer have my children full-time. I miss them. I love them. My greatest fear is realized—I have become my own parents. I am desperate and need to surrender.

Like waking up in a dry desert, I am thirsty for help. I feel lost and alone, so I drive to my mom and stepdad's house, desperate for answers. My mom is twenty-four years sober and my stepdad is twenty-nine. I can't lose my kids. I just can't.

I pull into their driveway and get out of the car with what little energy I have left. My mom greets me at the front door. I walk inside and crumple to the ground, crying, empty, and anguished.

My stepdad, Ross, looks at my mom. "Pat, can you please give us a minute?"

"Sure thing." She turns and heads to their bedroom.

I look at Ross, tears in my eyes. "I have a problem."

"We know, Serge. We are here to help you. But you have to want it. Do you want the help?" Ross asks me compassionately.

I know my level of despair is rock bottom. "If I don't get help, I will be dead in a week, guaranteed. I will keep looking for stronger drugs to numb this pain. I just don't care anymore."

"Let me make some phone calls. We need to get you into treatment."

Ross helps me to my feet. I can barely walk so I flop in the La-Z-Boy chair. I am lifeless and broken. And worst of all, I think, I have become my parents.

Ross and my mom give me a good dose of tough love. Ross always saw me as a son, and I am grateful for his role in my life. In a week, I am on my way to a treatment centre for addiction. It's four hours away from home, so I won't see my kids for a while. It breaks my heart. I love them so much. But if I am going to be the father who they need—who they deserve—treatment is necessary.

The addiction counsellor is stringent; he doesn't mess around. During my first group session, I try to blame others (like my parents) for my life. He stops me in my tracks. "We can spend all day blaming others, Serge, but I promise you won't feel any better. What you need to do is look at how you played a role in where you are today in your life."

What? I am shocked. How do I have anything to do with being in a treatment centre? It is clearly everyone else's fault.

"You need to forgive others," the counsellor continues. "Horrible things have happened to you in your life . . . I'm not ignoring that. But the longer you blame others, the longer you will stay sick and the quicker the disease of addiction will kill you. More than anything, you need to forgive yourself."

I start to cry uncontrollably.

"Your parents did the best they could with what they were given. They were sick, too."

My parents were sick? I let that resonate within the confines of my mind. The thought never occurred to me before.

"No parent is perfect, and some are downright bad. But from what I can tell, yours love you and want you to get well."

He's right. I am like my parents in some ways—and that's okay. I am sick just like they are, and I need help and I'm ready to accept it. I can become a better person if I stop blaming others for where I am in my life. My actions are my responsibility—and tomorrow I will be a better dad. I am not perfect—no one is—but I love my children with all my heart, and I want to be the best possible version of myself for them. What a wonderful gift recovery is. But one of the greatest gifts of all is that I finally love myself, too.

Serge Gagné grew up in a small town north of Sudbury, but now he is a heavy equipment operator in Barrie, Ontario. He has two kids and enjoys camping, fishing, and helping others with their recovery from addiction. He is living his life one day at a time.

Thanks for being apart
of this.
 Keep it simple!!

Serge Gagné

PART II
EVOLUTION

ev·o·lu·tion
[ev-uh-loo-shuh n]

the process of working out or developing

a process of continuous change from a lower, simpler, to a higher, more complex, or better state: growth

EVOLUTION

Ann Thomas

MY DAD TURNS EIGHTY-EIGHT this month, a mere seventeen days away. I need to call him and ask him a question. I dial his number automatically. I know it by heart. I doubt I am capable of forgetting it—the same number I memorized as a child. My parents haven't moved or changed their telephone number since before my birth, over fifty-one years ago.

"Hi Mom," I say. "Is Dad around?"

"No, he's chopping down a tree in the backyard."

This should be a surprise, but it's not—chopping trees, cutting grass, shovelling driveways, checking Facebook—all simply mundane everyday activities for my dad. He doesn't let a number stop him from doing the things he loves—learning, growing, evolving. What is surprising: I am asking for Dad. I usually talk to Mom.

"Can you have him call me when he gets in?"

"Sure thing," she answers.

Growing up, I didn't know a lot about my dad's childhood—or his own father for that matter. I knew Dad grew up in St. John's, Newfoundland, during the Second World War, and his father, Grandpa, as I knew him, looked like an older, more-weathered version of my own father. In contrast to my dad, Grandpa was missing half his index finger on his right hand, noticeable and mysterious. To Grandpa, sometimes it felt like the finger still existed, and he would reach for his tea and knock over the cup. To me, Grandpa was neither malice nor charisma; he was somewhat a non-entity. However, when observing my father in relationship to Grandpa, the neutrality was palpable, a combination of indifference and guard so calculated it appeared to be concealing something I did not yet understand.

Grandpa was my only living grandparent on my father's side when I was born. I remember visiting him in the long-term care facility occasionally. We drove from Oshawa to Hamilton—auto city to steeltown—a few times a year to see him. If there was little traffic in the parking lot, my dad would drive in the exit. I remember the anxiety welling up in me. "You shouldn't do that, Dad," I would say.

"No one's coming. It's fine," he would answer.

To him, it was harmless fun; to me, it was insolence. Following the rules, perfection, and utmost compliance were important to me. Maybe too important for a child, forming the background noise of anxiety that would follow me for many years, pushing me to weigh my worth based on achievement and pleasing those around me.

When we arrived, I would hear the voice of a sportscaster, commentating on the boxing match that always played on the TV in the lounge; I would notice the pungent smell wafting up from a tin of roll-your-own tobacco sitting beside the half-finished crossword puzzle in the daily newspaper on Grandpa's side table in his bedroom; and I would see the nameplate STANLEY THOMAS on his door. His complete name was actually Matthew Stanley Thomas, but his friends called him "Stan." Like the precision of a Swiss watch, we would bring chocolate liqueurs, a box of tobacco, and rolling papers every Christmas or birthday. "He likes his drink," my dad would mention.

As an adult, I am embarrassed to admit I liked visiting Grandpa, not because I felt particularly close to him, but rather because he would sometimes dispense five- or ten-dollar bills to my brother Doug and me. It was kind of hit and miss what amount would be given out, so the car ride held a type of unique anticipation.

The most remarkable memory I have of my grandpa was when, on one particular visit, we shared the news that I had begged and pleaded my way into owning a puppy. We were having a rather difficult time coming up with a suitable name for the furry bundle, who was a mysterious mix of breeds.

"Hmmm," Grandpa said. "Well, how about Oleo?"

"Why Oleo?" I asked.

"Oleo is a mixture of oils, and it sounds like your dog is a mixture of breeds."

That day Oleo was christened.

During the Christmas holidays when I was eleven, my oldest brother Dave took me to his wife's family cottage for a few days. Upon my return, my dad said to me, "You need to sit down, Ann."

My dad had never said that to me before. Even at eleven, I knew something was wrong. "Who died?" I asked.

"Grandpa."

I didn't cry. At least not that day. When my sister-in-law hugged me while, for the first time, I peered at a deceased body before the service started, I fought to maintain composure. It wasn't until a week later when I happened upon a stuffed animal in my toy box—a blue bear whom I had affectionately named Bluebeary—that I really cried. He was given to me by Grandpa.

I start supper—zoodles, spiralized zucchini with tomato sauce—making an inordinate number of dirty dishes. I am trying to follow a mostly-vegan-mostly-ketogenic-mostly-impossible diet. I remember to phone my parents again. Maybe Mom forgot to tell Dad to call.

"Hello." I hear my dad's voice. "I'll get your mother."

"Actually, I want to talk to you."

"Well, okay. What's new?"

"I am working on developing a new project. It will be a collection of stories about mental health."

"That sounds interesting," he responds.

Through the years as I grew into adulthood, nuances of the complicated relationship between my father and his own father would leak out, hue on hue, painting a more detailed picture with subtle gradation, offering insight into my dad's tactical dance between resentment and duty in affinity with his father.

Dad grew up in Newfoundland during the time when England claimed it as a British colony and before the time Canada called it a province. He was born in house number eight on Eric Street. It still stands today; I've checked Google Earth. The house rests on a hill. To be fair, most everything in St. John's sits on a hill, the city jutting both out and up from an unforgiving ocean harbour.

Measured in units of time, the Second World War was only decades ago; however, if measured by increments of change, the number would be infinite. It was a different world back then.

The residents of number eight consisted of my dad, his older sister, his machinist-father, his teacher-mother, and his grandfather and grandmother. In fact, the house was owned by his grandfather, a carpenter by trade.

St. John's was a hub for the war—blackouts at night, don't light a cigarette outside or leave the curtains undrawn—soldiers, sailors, airmen all the time, everywhere. The first floor of the house was rented out to a Canadian petty officer and his wife, originally from Hamilton.

For my dad, life was good despite the occasional fist fight with some of the tough kids at his inner-city school. My father was skinny and hardly a threat. But then, when my dad was eight, something changed with Grandpa, and to this day, my father has no idea why.

My grandpa began to drink and become abusive to his family. Friday nights—Friday was payday—he would bring home alcohol and magazines and newspapers, and after supper (quite often after a big argument with his wife), he would go to his tiny bedroom and frequently spend the weekend there, emerging only for meals.

On one occasion, Grandpa had a big fight with Grandma, and Great Grandpa Parsons could not endure it anymore. To get away from the tension, he started to walk the five miles to Mount Pearl Park where he had built a cottage. As he walked toward the cottage via the railway line, a train came. He was caught between a steep bank into the river and the tracks themselves. He also was somewhat hard of hearing. In any case, the iron handle of a freight car struck my great-grandfather just behind the ear, killing him.

My father's dog, a mutt named Chum—light brown with some white patches—existed in a leash-free bliss. He just did his own thing, ran loose, followed whomever he wished. At Great Grandpa Parson's funeral procession—horse and cart, mourners walking—Chum followed in line all the way to the cemetery. He was also sighted at the gravesite several weeks later.

Things did not improve: arguments at mealtimes, food thrown off the table, bad language, my grandmother's weekly stipend thrown through the kitchen door—just a humiliating and embarrassing situation. Yet, my dad remembers Grandpa being the kindest and most helpful, polite, and attentive person toward neighbours or strangers.

When he hit his teens, my dad started liking school, or at least some subjects in school: geometry, algebra, trigonometry, physics, and English. He also developed an irresistible attraction to anything that had a wire connected to it. Miraculously, he didn't electrocute himself.

Then he read in *Popular Mechanics* about crystal sets. So off to Mundy Pond he went. (His father said there was a man there who used to have a crystal set and he still might have a crystal. Turned out he didn't.) So my dad ordered some parts from ads in the magazine. He also figured out how to fashion an antenna. His family always had a ladder up to the roof of the two-storey house. Nobody challenged him as he went up the ladder, sat on the edge of the roof, and attached antenna wire that spanned from the roof down to his bedroom window. He did this many times as he experimented with different configurations. He could now listen to the radio whenever he wished. In fact, he had his headphones on, listening to a crystal set on August 5, 1945, when he heard the news of the first atomic bomb being dropped on Hiroshima.

After the war, a surrendered German U-boat was put on display in the St. John's Harbour, allowing many (including my father) the opportunity to tour its contents. A different era, indeed.

Time would pass and my dad would end up in Ontario, but eventually so would his father, always leaving a trail of challenges often complicated by his drinking.

"I think you should write a story," I suggest to my dad.

"Oh, really?"

"Yeah. You are a great writer, and I think it is so interesting when I hear about life in St. John's during the war."

"Well, what's the book about again?"

"Mental health," I remind.

"What would I write about? I don't really have any experience with mental illness."

A little surprised, I answer, "True, but what about your dad?"

"What about my dad?"

"He was an alcoholic, wasn't he?"

Hesitation. "Yeah."

"Addiction *is* a mental illness."

Radio silence.

Through the phone line, I feel the picture expand: lens focusing, depth of field defining, frame widening.

"I never thought of it that way before," he answers.

A shift so subtle yet seismic—deliberate and permanent—occurs, proving that evolution at any age is possible.

Ann Thomas is an observer of life and a reflective writer. She would very much like you to follow Wintertickle Press on Twitter @Wintertickle.

HIDING FROM CHILDREN
Autumn Aurelia

IT STARTS ON A FROSTY winter's morning when I am eight. My mother leaves me alone in the car for two minutes while she drops off a Christmas present to her friend.

"Stay in the car, Sam. Don't move. I'll be right back, okay?"

I smile and promise her I'll do just that. And I do. I sit and wait, but she doesn't return as quickly as she said she would. Something about being stuck in the car alone makes me feel afraid.

My breathing quickens, the boom-boom of my heart can be felt in my back, my legs, my chest; before I know it, I am standing outside the car.

Time passes slowly, and everything is hazy. But after a while, my mother appears behind me, furious. I have disobeyed her instructions. She is a cautious mother.

"Sam, what are you doing out of the car?" she pushes. But I have no answer for her. My body is frozen, my eyes fixated on the concrete beneath us.

"Sam, why aren't you answering me?" She follows my eyes toward the ground, and that's when she sees it.

"Sam, did you touch that needle?"

Disease equals death.

Did I touch the needle?

Disease equals death.

No, of course I didn't.

Disease equals death.

Did I use it?

Disease equals death.

Then I reply with the only answer I am sure of: "I don't know, Mum."

And so it begins: a life of doubt, danger, and darkness. I fear things that most children my age simply don't. I start to question everything, like if the waiter drugged my meal, or if I drank bleach instead of water. From that day forward, a voice appears in my head that was never there before. It is a man, of that much I am certain. I think that maybe I am hearing God, but the lady at Sunday School says that God is good, so I decide the voice inside my head is the devil. It takes nineteen years to find out that this devil is actually the workings of my own mind; this is the voice of obsessive-compulsive disorder (OCD).

You kiss your mum on the lips. Don't you think that's wrong, Sam? You're disgusting. It's a sin. You're going to hell.

My every minute is spent worrying, obsessing, and checking; and no one around me has a clue—not my mother, and certainly not my drunk, emotionally absent, and abusive father. To them, I am a carefree child who enjoys spending time alone in her room with her collection of toy ponies and teddy bears. All the while this hidden illness grows inside me like a tumour, gaining complete control of my brain.

I have a rather strange relationship with the devil, for he is neither bad nor good. Sure, he tells me that I have done awful, terrifying things I never remembered doing—or could never imagine doing—but he also protects me and those I love.

If you don't rub your hands together sixty-two times, your mum will die.

In my eyes, he is magic. If he tells me to do something, I will. And he never tells me to do bad things. They are always strange, odd behaviours that make me look a little silly, but if my actions save someone from death, what does it matter how peculiar they look?

As time goes on, however, his requests become incessant, infiltrating my every thought. He no longer wants me to rub my hands together sixty-two times, but instead one hundred and eighty-four. And it isn't just my mum that will die. He starts telling me stories about bus crashes and murders. He says if I don't perform these tasks for him, someone is going to get shot, or that a bus full of children will crash and everyone will die.

My mother watches the news constantly, and she is always crying for someone's missing child or for the victims of another school shooting. Little does she know I am the cause. The devil is working me too hard, and I can't possibly keep up with all of the things he asks of me.

At fourteen, things get more intense as I begin to experience flashbacks of sexual abuse I suffered as a child. I was eight when the abuse started—the very same time that the devil decided to take up residence in my mind.

The most difficult night of my life is the night I lose my mother's love, the night that the devil tells me I am pure evil. He isn't playing nice anymore.

Mum and I are lying side by side on her bed, just as we used to do most nights. Lights down low, the radio plays softly in the background while she caresses the tips of my hair, lovingly curling each piece around her long, painted fingernails.

For a very brief moment, the devil isn't there, and I am quite simply my mother's daughter, loved and cherished. Pure. For a moment, I remember what happiness feels like. But in my experience with mental illness, happiness does not last, and the road to darkness begins with one thought. One dark and dangerous thought has the ability to alter your entire life, and indeed it does.

"On tonight's show we're going to be tackling the topic of childhood abuse."

My mind tunes in a little louder to the radio. I wish it doesn't. It is a life-changing moment.

And then . . .

"Abused children can go on to abuse others," insists the host.

Frozen, I listen with fear and disgust. And the devil, he is back—louder, fiercer, more terrifying than ever before.

You're an abuser, Sam! You can't ever go near a child again.

My mother, still next to me, completely oblivious to the thoughts running through my head, tuts and sighs like she always does when something bothers her.

"Disgusting, Sam, isn't it? What kind of person would do such a thing?"

You will, Sam, says the devil. *You heard the man. Abused children go on to abuse others.*

Without saying a word to my mother, I quickly remove myself from the room. She can't witness this. She can't know that her only child is this sick, twisted monster who is destined to become a child abuser.

You're evil, Sam. Nobody can love you now. You have to stay away from children, do you hear me?

I hear him. I hear his panic, his fear, his urgency.

I will never go near a child again, I reply to him. *I'll stay away from children, I promise. I'm a monster. Oh, God! I'm so, so sorry. I promise I'll never ever go near a child. I won't. I won't.*

And your mum, you can't let her treat you like this anymore, do you hear me? You don't deserve her love, Sam. Can you imagine if she knew what you were? She'd abandon you in an instant.

From that day on, I reject all my mother's hugs. I become cold and detached, convincing myself I am, indeed, unlovable, that I am a sinner. And then, suddenly everything and everyone I once knew and loved becomes tainted, because I am tainted: a risk to children, an abuser in the making, an abomination, someone to be feared—killed even.

As I develop into a teenager, the devil becomes less of a thing living inside of my mind. Instead, I become one with him. These are *my* thoughts now, and that is far scarier than believing that someone else is responsible for them.

Days, weeks, months, and years go by, with my thoughts growing darker and more terrifying every waking moment. New obsessions present themselves at every given opportunity. I go from fearing I will snap my dog's neck one minute to believing that I had murdered someone without remembering it the next.

The four years I spend at university are among the most difficult, tortured years of my life. Each and every night, I lock myself away in my bedroom by dragging large pieces of furniture across the floor.

Cupboard in place? *Check.*

Desk in place? *Check.*

Chair in place? *Check.*

It seems logical to me that if I can't trust myself during my waking hours, I should be extra cautious while sleeping. What if I do something bad during the night and don't remember it?

With everything in place, all furniture pushed against the door, I feel a little safer that I won't "escape." This setup gives me a false sense of protection, acting as a barrier between my thoughts and the possible danger I believe myself to be.

Ashamed, I keep all of these thoughts and fears locked away from others, burying them deep within me, where no one will ever be able to find them.

But all of this becomes too much for me—the dark thoughts, the horrid fears, the lengths to which I will go to avoid children. Most painful, however, is the six- to eight-hour rituals of having to physically write out every child I have seen during the day just to check I haven't harmed anyone. Most nights I am awake until four or five o'clock, performing these rituals, crying myself into an uneasy and restless sleep.

Now, at twenty-eight years of age, I have had enough. This enduring battle with my mind will finally be over. Here I sit, cross-legged on the edge of my bed, medication of all kinds scattered around me, ready to die.

There's no way I can beat this thing, I think. *I'm done.*

But then, in a moment of calm, I reason with my mind and decide that before I send myself to such a final end, I will look online to see if there is some explanation for why I am so afraid of myself.

I go over to my desk, open up my laptop, and type into Google the words I have always been afraid of writing: I'm scared I will abuse children.

The search results direct me to an article published on the *Guardian* online by Rose Bretécher. The article outlines the reality of an illness called obsessive-compulsive disorder, or more specifically, in our cases, Pure O.

And just as the corners of my world folded in on me all of those years ago when I was fourteen, they finally unfold at twenty-eight years of age, and for the first time since it all began, I can see a spark of hope. At the very least, I know I am not alone. Tears of joy and sadness work their way through me that night as I recall years of obsessional thinking and compulsive behaviours. I cry for the child who never got to be a child, and for the ones who never knew what they were suffering from, the ones who tragically went on to kill themselves because they had no idea that they, too, were living with something that millions of us struggle with—something treatable.

Even though I find hope and solidarity, I know the road ahead won't be easy. I know managing symptoms and finding treatments will be works-in-progress. I know I may also suffer from other mental illnesses. I know the path to recovery is not linear. But I also know I am not alone, and in this moment I am still here. And with that, there is hope.

Autumn Aurelia spends her days working on her first novel, cuddling her furbabies, and campaigning for better mental health awareness. She is a long-term sufferer of obsessive-compulsive disorder, borderline personality disorder, post-traumatic stress disorder, and major depressive disorder. Autumn is the founder of *Inside The Bell Jar*—a literary journal that gives a voice to those who feel restricted by their own battles with mental illness. To learn more about her, visit autumnaurelia.com.

THE PRICE OF RICHES

Sarah Beth McClure

HE BRINGS ME THREE DOLLARS and forty-seven cents from his piggy bank and asks, "Will that get us to Disney World?"

For months, he has been talking about this magical place and his dream to one day walk those sacred pathways, leading to every character he's ever loved. He's four years old, and our daughter is five—their imaginations are still magical, but the hourglass of untamed beliefs is losing sand faster than I can keep up. It's an opportunity to watch their faces light up with unparalleled enchantment; surely to miss it would leave scars on my soul.

I choose my words carefully. "We just don't have the money right now, bud. One day, I hope we will get there."

I haven't worked in over a year; and the year before that, the business I stubbornly swore would be our ticket to riches . . . well, it bankrupted and plummeted us so far into debt that I sometimes wonder if we will ever walk without chains tightening around our necks. Somehow, every necessary bill gets paid and every meal is served hot on the kitchen table; it blows my mind every week. Our lifestyle was demolished when our income was cut in half; the adjustment from that has been close to unbearable—but humbling at the same time. Our house is warm and the mortgage is paid. We have food in our bellies, running water to drink, and more love than can be contained within our own family.

I have children who think I hung the moon and a warrior husband who has climbed out of the rubble with me and has chosen to remain loyal even though I blew his world apart. We have been stripped bare of our recognizable life, but our souls have been refined in a way that isn't possible unless you survive a fire of epic proportions. We are the lucky ones because we are still standing, albeit naked and on shaky ground. I am more thankful for the financial chains around our necks than I ever was for all the material possessions we took for granted. With every successful bill payment, I am reminded that miracles truly happen, and it's a constant celebration that we survived another month.

I stand in front of my son with his outstretched hand, secretly blaming myself. There are even worse days when shame wraps a cage around my bed where I wallow in grief and resentment for all the Disney dream vacations I see on Facebook. I can't hop on a plane and take my kids to the most magical place in the world. I can't give them that one rite of passage that every child should take. But they have never given up hope, and any loose change they find is placed in their piggy banks or the Disney savings plate on the kitchen counter. They still believe their parents carry magic in their wallets and that, come hell or high water, we will get them there—and so they patiently wait.

I know what you're thinking, because the normal side of me is thinking the same thing: I should find a job. Simple answer. It makes complete sense, right? I'm qualified, and I have truly wrestled with the idea for months now. I obtained a bachelor's degree, and I worked a successful and well-paying career for nearly ten years before my life imploded. I'm not bragging; those credentials played a part in ultimately breaking my soul.

You see, my spirit hid a ticking time bomb from me—and everyone else around me. By maintaining complete and utter control of my life and the lives around me, I managed my condition without even realizing how miserable it was making me. Looking back, the evidence of bipolar disorder is so apparent that I can't believe how blind I remained for thirty-two years. The people close to me still question if I truly suffered from the disorder my whole life—but that's because the control I maintained hid the toxic thoughts that I ignored daily. I coped and self-medicated when necessary, the dosage just enough to keep my sanity. Then I got married, gave birth to two beautiful children within a fourteen-month time span, and continued working and self-proclaiming myself as supermom. Then I was laid off from my job, a job I enjoyed with people I loved dearly. Of course, this was my moment to purchase and build a business that would make us millionaires. Private jet to Disney World whenever we wanted. That was the crossroads where I stepped onto a looming path that was screaming for me to run far away and never return, but my stubbornness is toxic.

I lost control. I lost complete control and fell off the saddle; bipolar disorder was there waiting and laughing as it stole the reins. I can still hear it mocking me, "Buckle up, Buttercup." Essentially, my disorder spurred the horse and rode straight toward a spiralling and endless vortex of mania, leaving the controlling version of me face down in the mud.

What I didn't realize at the time was my sudden money spending, binge drinking, and irrational thinking was a textbook case of a manic episode. A very intense episode that I had never experienced previously, because bipolar only ran along beside me, my control blocking the reins. I was spiralling upward and increasingly out of control with nothing to stop me besides complete and total self-destruction. I became a person that I didn't recognize. I stared at this second version of myself in the mirror every day, and she seemed fun and the life of the party. However, my heart knew that she was not someone I wanted to know—still, this strangely curious girl laughed and pleaded that I keep spinning with her. I devastated many people along that twisted and dysfunctional path—the amount of damage is unfathomable.

And then I fell, and I fell hard. I fell into the deepest pits of depression one could ever face, and I continued spiralling downward as quickly and intensely as I had spiralled up. Bipolar depression is different, and it is deep. It takes root at rock bottom and grows around its victims, making the potential escape almost impossible. Those who make it become warrior fighters that never give up, ever.

This new and depressed version of me was colourless and rarely spoke. She detested sunshine or relationships, and she wanted me dead—she nearly succeeded. She held me hostage inside the walls of my house, and her branches quickly grew around me, tightening their grasp as they staked their claim on my life. She chained me to my bed, then she whispered continuously in my ear that I was worthless and only made the lives of those around me miserable. I hurt people. It's what I did. They didn't deserve it, but she didn't care, and she would continue with those swirling thoughts until I ended my life. She told me it was the only escape.

Luckily, my children kept me alive during that time. I spent what small amount of energy I had on making sure they were fed and safe. The thought of not seeing them grow up and the incurable pain they would feel if I was not at their graduations and weddings gave me just enough strength to grasp the edge of a cliff and hold on until my husband and family could ensure my medication was beginning to release the grip the branches of depression had over my entire body. My children have grown into incredible little humans who have learned the art of forgiveness and self-sufficiency at a young age, partly because of my illness.

Fear is the reason my resumé remains the same as it did ten years ago. Rationally, I know we need more income immediately, but if I choose this route, will the pressure push me over the edge again? Could I destroy my family by getting swept into another upward spiral? Could I survive another downward spiral?

My children deserve a trip to Disney World more than most—they've earned it. It would be a small reward compared to the battle I would have lost without them and their understanding and forgiving hearts. But I cannot give them that reward if it means I'm stolen from their lives again. I vowed that mania and depression would never mother my children ever again.

As I look at my son and his offering of three dollars and forty-seven cents, I wrestle with the decision between taking side jobs just to make ends meet or full-time work so we can take an extravagant lifestyle for granted again. I just cannot stop leaning toward the side of miracles and the celebration of bill payments being made. I cannot help but have faith that the magic those kids believe lives in our pockets will someday miraculously manifest. Maybe our pockets really are magical . . . if we choose to believe!

Sarah Beth McClure is a wife, mother, daughter, sister, friend, and warrior. She is also a recovering people-pleaser. Humour is her favourite medicine; and she's an advocate for mental health, suicide awareness, and removing the stigma surrounding these issues. She is also an aspiring bestselling author, even though she still hasn't started her first book . . . stay tuned. You can follow her blog at sarahbethmcclure.com. With the generosity of friends, Sarah Beth McClure and her family did finally make it to Disney World!

RIVERS SHALL FLOW

Marleah Atlookan

A VOICE TRAILS AFTER ME in the main hallway of Dryden High School: "Marleah."

I turn to see Ms. McMonagle, the school's graduation coach, power walking toward me.

"Hi Ms. McMonagle," I answer. I like her, as far as adults go. She isn't a teacher, exactly. She has a classroom where we can go to hang out sometimes, and there are always snacks there. Her job is to track and help students who may be at risk of not graduating. She seems to get us, partly—maybe—because she is Métis.

"Marleah," she repeats, "I have a proposition for you. There is a board meeting at the school next week, and we are looking for some students to cater the event. Of course, I thought of you to lead this."

Secretly, or maybe not so secretly, I want to become a chef when I grow up.

"Sure," I answer, avoiding eye contact and pulling my arms up into my long sleeves.

"But," and then comes the condition, "if you don't show up for classes, you can't do it."

I know why she is saying this. When I can get away with it, I skip classes. I experience a lot of anxiety, and it is hard to concentrate. I want to finish high school, but sometimes the prospect of it is very daunting.

When I was five years old, we returned one night to our northern home at Eabametoong First Nation, also known as Fort Hope. I saw my mother's body hanging from a pipe overhead. It was scary and sad. I couldn't understand how someone who was supposed to love me could do this. She was so important to my brothers and me. She didn't die that day, but she suffered severe brain damage and died ten years later while living in a care facility. She choked on some food just last year. It is hard to focus on math or civics when your mind wanders to the events of your past.

But I know that what Ms. McMonagle is asking isn't unreasonable.

"That's fair," I answer.

"You will have to draw up grocery lists, find the best deals, and put together the menu for each monthly meeting."

I am up to the task. In fact, I am excited.

After my last class, I am eager to go home and get started on preparing a menu.

"Hi Dad," I say as I open the door. He is on the couch, watching TV—the living room is his bedroom. He sleeps there so both my brother and I can have our own rooms. My dad moved to Dryden from Lac Seul after my mom's suicide attempt and took my brother and me into his care. He felt that leaving the reserve would allow us to have better access to health and education services. He is a survivor of residential schools and never talks to us about what happened. I often wonder what *his* childhood was like.

I go into my room and flop onto my bed. I take out my phone to text my best friend Titanice: Guess what?

What?

Ms. McMonagle asked me to head up catering for the school board meetings!!!!

No way. Really? U must be excited.

Ya, it should be fun, I answer.

I look up at the flag on the wall behind my bed: a canoe between two teepees. It represents my people—the Eabametoong, who are part of the Ojibway Nation of the Nishnawbe-Aski.

The teepee on the left is black and represents our forefathers and present-day people who have gone before us. The red canoe in the centre represents the living blood of the Eabametoong Nation of today. The white teepee on the right symbolizes the Great Spirit, who has guided us, and will continue to guide us, through our life's journey. The backdrop to the flag is three horizontal stripes: yellow, green, and blue, from top to bottom. Each colour stands for something different: yellow for as long as the sun shall shine, green for as long as the grass shall grow, and blue for as long as the rivers shall flow.

What should I make for the first meeting? I text.

Hmmm. I dunno, she answers.

I think and write back, What about pork loin? Or maybe a rack of lamb?

That sounds complicated lol, Titanice answers.

I can also do lasagna, salad, and tacos . . .

That sounds good.

The following week is filled with planning, shopping, organizing, bossing other kids around, and my favourite thing—cooking.

It is so much fun. My time is filled, and my mind is focused. I also attend classes regularly.

The day of the board meeting comes, and I am busy preparing. The only thing my mind has room for is the task at hand.

"I'm keeping a watchful eye on you and your team," Ms. McMonagle tells me.

I giggle. "You don't have to."

"You seem to be enjoying yourself," she observes.

"I am," I reply.

"You will make a great executive chef in a restaurant one day." She smiles.

The meal is a big success. Everybody loves the food, and I get lots of compliments. I feel . . . proud. It is a night I will never forget. It feels almost magical. I go home, say hello to my dad and to my brother, and right before I head into my room, my dad asks, "How was it?"

"Good," I reply. "Really good. I think the reason I like it so much is because when I am cooking, I am so busy preparing a dish, and that is the only thing I can think about in that moment. I have to concentrate on the task at hand, and I can't think about . . . other things."

My dad nods, knowingly.

"Goodnight," he says.

"Goodnight, Dad," I say. I go to my room, thankful for a quiet mind and a tired body. I reflect on what an awesome day today has been. I realize that it is easier to focus on "other things" when I actually *have* other things in my life to focus on. In this moment, I vow to find and pursue those activities that will fuel my passion, ignite my concentration, and propel me forward— for as long as the sun shall shine, for as long as the grass shall grow, and for as long as the rivers shall flow.

Marleah Atlookan is a student, a daughter, a friend, and an aspiring chef. She is a member of the Eabametoong Nation and resides in Northern Ontario.

MY RELATIONSHIP WITH CATS

H.A. Fraser

PAIN ATTACKS ME IN MY deepest sleep. I feel the incredible choking pressure on my chest. Breathing is a labour. *Oh. My. Goodness. I am having a heart attack.*

The reason I know without a doubt that I am having a heart attack isn't because I am some type of medical expert. No, the reason I am keenly aware of the symptoms of a heart attack is because my husband, Jack, suffers from anxiety, and when it bubbles over, it manifests physically. It feels as if I have taken him to the emergency department in every city we have ever visited. That may be a little bit of an exaggeration, but not much. I have heard doctor after doctor explain, while poring over Jack's perfect ECG record, that, with an actual heart attack, there is often a tightness of the chest; some people describe it as a great weight pressing mercilessly against them. And that is exactly what I am experiencing at this particular moment. The weight on my chest is heavy, pressing, and I am having difficulty breathing. My mind wanders, and I start questioning. *Is this the day I die? Is this how I die? I am only fifty years old. Why now?*

I remember the first trip we took out to Prince Edward Island. The night before we were to fly home, Jack woke up in a panic.

It was two a.m. and I was tired. Really tired. We were flying home the next morning, and I simply wanted to sleep. In fact, I was of the opinion that I needed to sleep.

"I think I should go to the hospital," he said.

I sighed. Loudly. I stumbled out of bed, found my jeans, and reluctantly pulled my crumpled sweatshirt over bed-head hair. I was always plagued with niggling doubt that maybe this time it really was something serious.

"Okay, let's go."

Charlottetown at two a.m. is pretty quiet. The kind doctor on duty thoroughly examined Jack. Wisely reading the situation, the physician asked, "Could you possibly be worried about anything?"

Jack does not like to fly. And by that, I mean he is absolutely shit-scared of flying. We usually have to drug him to even get him on a plane. I remember him being barely conscious after a flight to the U.K. The meds hadn't worn off and coherence eluded him. At Heathrow, an intimidating and incredibly busy airport, the customs officer asked, "Where are you headed in the U.K.?" Instead of mentioning our destination, Jack answered, "Two weeks."

So, yes, the Charlottetown doctor had definitely read the situation. Jack answered, "Well"—slight pause—"we are flying back home tomorrow."

"You don't like to fly?" he queried. "Are you thinking about it, possibly worrying?"

"No, I'm not really thinking about it much."

My tired eyes glared at him. *Are you serious?*

Jack continued, "Well, I don't like flying, and I really am not looking forward to it. Maybe that is playing on my mind . . . a little bit."

Now four a.m., we piled into the rented car and headed back to the bed and breakfast in an outlying area. I knew that we would have to get up in two hours and drive back this same route. We didn't speak, and I sighed again and again . . . and again.

I have seen the commercials. I know what I am supposed to do for a heart attack. I need to chew an Aspirin, or is it two? I know where they are—under the sink in the cupboard in the bathroom. I need to will myself awake, go to the bathroom, get two Aspirin, and chew them. *Why won't my eyes open? Please make my eyes open.*

Then there was that small town in cottage country when they had to phone and wake up the doctor on call at home to come in. The nurse set up the ECG and monitored Jack as we waited almost an hour for the physician to travel in.

It was our first day of vacation, and again, I had fallen into a deep, relaxing sleep, not eager to be interrupted or spend my night at the local hospital. But I found myself, yet one more time, listening intently to what a heart attack feels like. It was concluded that this possibly was a pulled muscle in the shoulder area, probably incurred while doing some heavy lifting the day prior.

I am still unconscious, but I can feel awareness of the real world increasing. I can now tell that I am lying on my back. The terrible pain in my chest is more than just pressure now. I can feel sharp stabs as well. It is so intense. I desperately need to open my eyes. *Open your eyes, Helen, damn it!*

Then there was the time when I was working as a wedding photographer, shooting a wedding about a fifty-minute drive from home. I was in the middle of photographing the bridal party getting ready when my cell rang. It was Jack.

"I need to go to the hospital."

We shared a vehicle, and I had it with me.

"I can't really help you right at this moment," I answered.

"But I need to go *now*."

Firmly I replied, "Jack, I am in the middle of photographing someone's wedding, a day that will hopefully occur only once in their lifetime. What exactly do you want me to do?" I didn't have time for a lengthy discussion. "Never mind. I will see if my friend can take you."

Irritation had escalated to resentment mixed with a little anger. I called a good friend and asked her to drive him to the hospital. She was just about to head in the other direction to drive two hours to visit her parents; however, she sensed the desperation in my pleas.

"I'll take him, but I can't wait around for him. I will have to leave him there."

I thanked her. It would have to do.

A few hours later, in a break after the ceremony, I called Jack. He was back at home. He was fine, and, thankfully, nothing was physically wrong. However, he forgot to bring his wallet and didn't have money for a taxi. He didn't have a way to get back, so he walked. It was about an eight-kilometre trek.

This is life and death, Helen. Open your eyes. Find and chew an Aspirin. Then call 9-1-1. You can do this. I am able to slightly pry my cement eyelids open. It feels like I am manually raising a heavy drawbridge with chains and gears, cranking hard to move even a millimetre at a time. Then, my eyelids shift a little more, and finally I cross the moat into the land of awake. I do not expect what happens next. It is the furthest thing from my mind. I find myself staring into the yellow-green eyes of my spawn-of-Satan cat, who is standing on my chest, glaring at me, nonchalantly, as if to say, "What's your problem?" To her disappointment, I gently remove her, and miraculously all my heart attack symptoms cease immediately.

Before now, when I looked at my husband's anxiety, I saw a cute little five-pound kitten sitting on his chest. What's all the fuss? It couldn't be that bad. However, in his mind, he was experiencing a fatal heart attack. How scary would that be? How awful it must be to really—and I mean *really*—believe that you are about to die. What must that feel like?

My stirring disturbs his sleep, and Jack sits up and mutters, "I don't feel right."

What I do next isn't nearly as remarkable as what I don't: I don't sigh loudly; my eyes don't roll, annoyed; no irritated comments are spewed. Instead I simply say, "I'm here. I'm sorry this is happening to you. Tell me how you feel."

Although I didn't have a heart attack that night, there was an attack on my heart. An arrow dipped in a small puddle of sympathy and understanding was cleverly, quickly, and skilfully slung into the centre of my being, shattering a layer of prejudice and stigma. I became a little more sensitive that night, and it is the catalyst for me to encourage Jack to seek professional help. He does, and life is so much better—for both of us.

The author William S. Burroughs once wrote, "My relationships with my cats has saved me from a deadly, pervasive ignorance."

If he only knew . . .

H.A. Fraser is a Canadian writer and the author of *Thank You, Yes Please*, a gratitude journal. You can find out more about H.A. Fraser's book by visiting thankyouyesplease.com.

BUTTERFLY

Heather Down

I AM NOT A NATURAL hugger. It just isn't in my nature. I respect and adore personal space, and I loathe those awkward moments when I don't know what is the most socially acceptable course of action. Is now a good time to shake someone's hand, or is a pat on the shoulder better; or is shaking hands what is called for? It is actually a standing joke among my closest friends. I remember when, after an extremely long run with our local run-club members, one guy decided to give each and every one of our sweaty crew a hug. Apparently, my expression gave my inner disdain away, and my two friends who witnessed the event couldn't stop laughing.

It is almost ten o'clock at night when I drop my daughter-in-law off, and my son greets us at the car door in the parking lot outside their four-storey apartment building.

"Hi," I say. "How are you doing?"

He is stepping side to side, glancing left and right, his agitation palpable.

"Not good. I left work today. I had to walk away or I don't know what I would have done."

Jason's speech is punctuated with expletives.

"What happened?" I ask.

"It's my supervisor. I can't stand the guy. Honestly, I thought I was going to punch him. I don't want to lose my job, and I don't want to go to jail for assault."

"Walk me through it," I say, trying to get a better feel for what happened. My son works solely on commission at a furniture shop.

"My numbers are down, and they called me in for a meeting. They asked me what was going on, and I said that I am having a bad time, a bad day . . ."

I know what he is talking about. On one hand, I am sad, as I know why he is having a difficult time, yet on the other hand, something inside me stirs to life as I realize at least Jason is talking, which is the first step.

"What did your supervisor say?"

"He said, 'We all have bad days, I have a bad day, so-and-so has a bad day.'"

"Oh. He should *not* have said that. I am so sorry."

"Mom, he has *no* idea. None. I'm not talking my-wife-is-pissed-off-at-me-because-I-didn't-take-the-garbage-out bad day . . . I held my dead child in my arms. That's not something you can just get over. I am depressed. Potential customers walk in and I literally run away from them. I can't handle the depression in addition to the stress of work. It's just too much."

"I agree. It's a lot, Jason. Are you talking to anybody?"

It had been six months since the stillbirth; the ominous butterfly donning the name tag on their hospital birthing-room. Twenty-two weeks; their second such loss. The first was earlier along and deemed a miscarriage, but when a woman gets beyond the nineteen-week mark, it is different. This was an eight-hour labour and a beautifully formed little boy with perfect features. I watched my son hold his own lifeless son, Jaymison. It didn't seem real, and in some ways, still doesn't. I held him, too. So many arrangements, but not the ones they were planning on. Baby showers, decorating the nursery, and purchasing a crib were replaced with death certificate, body pickup, cremation, and visits to the funeral home.

Jason had been the perfect husband, holding the baby first until Mirada warmed to the idea. He knew she would regret it if she didn't. He looked after her as best he could, but he didn't— or *couldn't*—talk. Not to her, not to anyone. Until he was ready to talk. Until the crack in the armour was too big to mask with the metaphorical dingy duct tape he was hoping would work.

Until today.

"I can't do it. I can't work and deal with this. I am not sleeping. At all. For months."

"Of course, Jason. Of course. Let's get you to the doctor and figure out how we can help you. You are going to have to talk in order to process this trauma."

"I know." He pauses. "I am ready."

And with that I drive home, my mind wandering back almost twenty-five years.

When I was twenty-six years old, I was an elementary school teacher at a small country school. I taught Grades 7 and 8 and wasn't much of a fan of the younger students. One day, while I was on yard supervision, an eight-year-old boy went rushing past me into a restricted area where they were digging up the old septic system. It wasn't safe.

"Get back here!" I yelled in my most authoritative voice. Didn't matter. The wiry blond boy ignored me and dodged and ducked his way around mounds of dirt. He alluded my chase.

I was furious. When the bell went, I marched into the vice-principal's office and told her to get that kid down to the office NOW!

"Calm down, Heather," she said as she put her hand on my shoulder.

I thought she was being condescending until she continued: "He and his two sisters have just come back from court. Their parents relinquished their rights and they are Crown wards. They are up for adoption."

I am floored . . . and totally, utterly in love. Six months later, I had three beautiful children. Talk about taking your work home with you! Jason, my son, is the oldest.

Jason can't get in to see his own doctor right away, so I take him to a local clinic the next day. We wait, and wait, and wait some more, making small talk and passing time.

A nurse calls us into the exam room. She is so pleasant and helpful.

"Ah, I see you have my sons' names. I have one son with your first name and another with your second."

Serendipitous, indeed.

"What brings you here?"

"I can't function at work, and it is so stressful. I am depressed. We had a stillbirth, and I held my dead child . . ."

He continues to leak out his story, one little detail at a time. It is difficult to watch your child, even if he is thirty-four years old, in so much pain. I do my best, but tears periodically escape my left, then right eye in random and unpredictable patterns.

"You certainly have reason to be depressed, Jason. You have experienced a very traumatic event, one that not a lot of people have experienced."

Then he delivers the crux of his worry. "I can't deal with the stress of the loss and the stress of work at the same time. I need time to get better, but I don't want to be fired. I can't cope with the financial stress in addition to everything else that I am going through."

The nurse replies with words I'll never forget—the words that will change my hug aversion for life: "They can't fire you for being *sick*."

His demeanor changes instantly and so does mine. Being believed, being acknowledged, and knowing that others realize that mental health is just that—health—is affirming. Just like physical health, mental health consists of wellness and sickness.

I don't remember much else that happens after that. A doctor comes in; a letter for work is written. Somehow time passes while I remain vaguely aware of my surroundings.

Upon leaving, I see the nurse by the front desk. I don't even remember her name. I do not question social norms or appropriateness or hesitate in any manner. I just find myself involuntarily enveloping her completely in my arms and whispering, "Thank you. Thank you so much."

Heather Down is a writer who has contributed stories and articles to over fifty magazines, including *Reunions* and *Guide*. She is the author of *A Deadly Distance* and *Postcards from Space: The Chris Hadfield Story*, both available on Amazon.

ZERO

Michelle Sertage

EATING IS HARD WHEN THE weight of your flaws looks like thirty extra pounds in the mirror. They say that my eyes are morphing my body into something it's not. I think to myself that if I could do that, I'd be skinny by now. I don't say this out loud; in fact, I have been hesitant to say anything at all. Being here is like being under arrest with no lawyer. Everything that comes out of my mouth can and will be used against me in a court of doctors, no doubt. They will do anything to keep me locked up for longer than I need to be, their little human test subject, I swear. At least that's what I think. They say I'm sick, that my thoughts are tainted by an intruder who will not stop until my heart does.

Thirty-five beats per minute, thirty-four, thirty-three . . .

A cold coin pressed on my chest, a gentle voice telling me to take deep breaths. As she lowers the stethoscope, the eyes of the nurse meet mine. I recognize that look—like she is searching for something; like my eyes are a puzzle to solve. She asks me if I am dizzy, tells me that my heart is sleepy today. I shake my head, absent-mindedly. I am now focused on clenching my stomach muscles. I heard somewhere that if you do it enough, you will start to see clearly defined abs. I can feel the food I'm forced to ingest pooling at my midsection, threatening to balloon out to a physique most accurately represented by the Pillsbury Doughboy. With the compulsory high calorie-fat-salt-carb meals I'm fed and the authoritative voices warning me to not-move-a-muscle, the ab clenching is more and more necessary every day.

The nurse brings me back to reality, telling me she will soon return with my lunch. I try to smile and fail. Those muscles have grown weaker than my will to survive. Giving me an empathetic look, the nurse lays her warm, smooth hands on top of mine. I watch as a frown crosses her face; my hand is as cold and lifeless as a corpse. She quickly leaves.

Death makes people uncomfortable.

It wasn't always like this. I used to be vibrant and adventurous. I used to eat pizza and popcorn on Friday nights with my family, with extra energy to see friends and make people laugh. Somewhere along the line, a perfect storm of events spun together in a giant hurricane of self-loathing, perfectionism, and fear. The aftermath was an apple for dinner one night and a rice cake the next. Although I was starving, it wasn't food I was hungry for; it was control. Everything was chaos, but at least I knew I was the one deciding to bring the fork to my mouth, or the one deciding not to. And so, I didn't.

Fading away is easy to do when done correctly. First, you eat a little healthier, maybe denying a dessert here or there. It will feel powerful. Maybe you walk for twenty minutes after dinner. Soon the twenty minutes will become thirty, forty, one-hour walks, then runs. The dessert-denier inside you turns into a carb-denier, then a dinner-denier; and suddenly you are fuelling your two-hour runs with a couple of baby carrots. You haven't responded to your friends' calls in over a month, and they have stopped trying. You will think it's better this way, that they could never understand you. And in all fairness, they don't. No one does. That's why you're here under these fluorescent hospital lights watching a nurse bring a tray of microwaved food to your bedside table.

Food is medicine, the doctors tell me. I repeat this mantra as I study the plate in front of me. The more I think about how this meal will soon be littering the confines of my small, pink stomach, the more I am revolted. Food is medicine? To me, mealtimes are war. Food is the weapon, meant to destroy me from the inside out. The voice in my head screams at me every time I lift up the fork.

LAZY! FAT! SLOB!

Halfway through the meal, a sense of defeat overwhelms me, and I burst into tears. I need the voice to be quiet, even if just for a minute. The nurse urges me to keep eating, tells me I'm doing well. I continue to sob uncontrollably, unable to go on. The nurse sighs and picks up the tray. As she is about to walk out the door, she turns to face me.

"You know, the more nourishment you give your body, the more nourishment you will get out of life. Think about all the beautiful experiences you have had. If you don't allow yourself to eat, the possibility of a beautiful future will be taken away. Be strong and fight for your life."

Her words linger, as she knew they would. It is in this moment I realize that the looming threat of death doesn't scare me. That is precisely why I don't eat. I want to disappear. Size zero, zero calories, zero pounds, zero life.

No, I am not scared to die.

Maybe, in fact, I am scared to live.

Michelle Sertage is a twenty-three-year-old who, because of her love of novelty and travel, calls herself a citizen of the world. She currently resides in Barrie, Ontario, where she studies holistic nutrition. Her hope is to be the healer she needed in her time of illness.

GRATITUDE

Natalie Harris

AWAKE ALL NIGHT. TOSSING AND turning. Not in a bad way. It is
like Christmas Eve. I finally succumb to the fact that sleep and
I are not friends, so I sit up and open my curtains to a dark hospital parking lot and look. I have time—more time—to just be,
to just sit, to just accept, to just breathe. I notice the spiders are
gone. In every room I've stayed in, there is always one spinning a
web in the corner of the window. Maybe they are gone because
it looks chilly outside (I can tell by the steam leaving the rooftop
pipes) . . . but I don't know for sure. I haven't felt the temperature outside for a week. Or maybe they are gone because they
don't need to be here anymore. I am going home, and the home
I watched them spin for days doesn't need to be watched anymore.

After a while of just looking outside, I get up and walk down
the quiet nighttime hall to find the clock at the nurses' station. Careful not to wake up a fellow patient who is asleep in a
chair—for fear that she may begin her sad, relentless pay-phone
calls too early—I walk in my socked feet and look at the time,
which has been so hard for me to keep track of for the last seven
days: 5:46 a.m. Okay, more time to wait. Getting a bit restless,
I take down the poster on my wall by carefully peeling off the

hospital stickers I used to adhere it. I roll it up and wonder if I will ever look at it again. Probably not—too many memories. Then I walk back and forth in my room, a place that, in a matter of days, went from feeling like jail to feeling like freedom, and I appreciate every step. In fact, I appreciate everything: my bed, my washroom, my window, and a few books. I don't need much to be okay.

With my mind too busy, I decide to try to read for a while, but I still can't focus. Is the sun finally starting to rise or is it still the streetlight's glow—and me willing it to be daytime? Finally, I hear a knock at the door. A new smiling face introduces himself as my nurse. This is wonderful! In my clock-less room, I now know that it is almost eight o'clock! Time for my medications and almost time to go home.

The nurse asks me, "Do you have anything in the hospital safe?" I reply, "I don't know." Then, "Do you have belongings at the nurses' station?" Once again, I answer, "I don't know." This is a loud reminder that I am unable to recall my first two days here. It stings a bit. I'm not going to lie. But as time goes by, I get used to saying why I am here. The word "overdose" rolls off my tongue with a strange ease.

I brush my teeth and decide to treat myself to one last fresh face cloth that is waiting for me in the hall—all my face cloths at home are waiting to be washed. I start to pack. It doesn't take long. One grocery bag and I am done. And I am finally able to trade my pyjamas for jeans!

My nurse peeks his head in the door. "Do you want to have your breakfast?" The residents of the floor are slowly waking. I walk down the hall to lots of good mornings from now-familiar faces. I find my tray on the table in the dining room, which is odd. I usually find it on the tall rack with everyone else's. Hmm, maybe this is what they do on the day you go home—like a special celebration. Probably not. More likely my place on the rack has been taken. Replaced by another new face who will most likely be scared and wary to walk into the dining room, just as I was at first. Days ago, I didn't want anyone to recognize me. I was a professional. I didn't belong here! They'd made a horrible mistake. But now the room is so easy for me to enter, because after a lot of soul-searching (and slowly swallowing my pride), I realize with all my heart that I do belong here.

I contemplate high-fiving or hugging every patient when I leave, but I decide that action might land me another week in Hotel Mental Health, so I don't. But I hope they feel my gratitude for their non-judgmental acceptance of me in my farewells—for becoming my intriguing, entertaining, and caring family for the week. I wonder when they will be going home. Or if they ever will. Or if they even have a home to go to.

So, as I wait for my boyfriend to walk through the door, I decide to look out the window and enjoy my cereal and shot of apple juice and be grateful. The web that was so beautifully woven for me caught me. I love you.

P.S. I am leaving this pen on the side table, as it was given to me by a fellow patient. This is an object that was once viewed as dangerous and not allowed to be in my possession only days ago. How's that for a reality check?

Natalie Harris is the celebrated author of *Save-My-Life School* and *Daily Lessons from Save-My-Life School*. You can follow her blog at paramedicnatsmentalhealthjourney.com.

FIRE

Tim Grutzius

ON THE OUTSIDE, I AM a firefighter. On the inside, I often battle a different kind of fire, the fire of my uncontrollable temper.

The car behind us is tailgating. I feel the emotion rising; not a slow, irritating anger, but rather a sudden, unexpected rage like gas on a bonfire. I slow down to antagonize the driver even more. "That'll teach them . . ." I say. I can feel my wife's eyes roll.

There is a break in the traffic on the highway, and the tailgater swerves around us. I speed up. I think I hear a sigh over the sound of our car's now-booming motor.

The speedometer climbs. I am doing 90 mph, trying to outgun the other driver.

I feel a sharp jab to my shoulder. I momentarily snap out of my engrossing trance, my focus shifting.

"Hey buddy, slow down! Not everything you drive is big, red, and has lights and sirens!" Judy half shouts at me.

I plug back into the reality of the situation and realize I am putting myself, and more importantly, Judy, in danger. I slow down and drive normally again.

My thoughts immediately go to shame and regret. I have mastered the art of self-deprecation, although my negative ruminations never seem to change my future reactions. I'm such an idiot. I could have killed us both. Judy deserves some-one better.

I chalk up my actions—or *reactions*, rather—to my upbring-ing. In my childhood household, impatience was a virtue, and according to this measuring stick, my parents were very virtuous, indeed! I grew up surrounded by a constant cloud of frustration and tension. I always assumed this was the root of my temper.

I wish today's reaction was an isolated incident, but it's not. There are so many to think about, but my mind wanders back to when I was twenty-four years old and my family had a cocker span-iel named Coco: "Could someone let that dog outside?" I remem-ber yelling to anyone within earshot. No one in the house moved.

I had let her out at least six times in the past half hour. She was barking incessantly.

I had experienced enough. The anger overtook me. Fist met wall and wall won, leaving my hand broken.

Since then, it doesn't matter where, and I certainly can't predict when, my irritation overcomes me. It can be anything, really: restaurants, assembling pool ladders, driving, interacting with colleagues at work.

At home, I can get unbearable.

"Come on, Vino," my wife says to our dog, "Tim's being an asshole again. Let's go upstairs." And with that, they go up to the bedroom, leaving me with the company of my temper.

Sometimes I bang my head against the wall, literally; the physical pain distracts me from my emotional distress.

I find myself at work when a flyer jumps out at me on our bul-letin board. It is only a standard-sized piece of paper, small in area but large in impact: INTRODUCTION TO FIREFIGHTER BEHAVIORAL HEALTH.

I am drawn in. It is a one-day workshop; however, it is being held too far away for me to attend.

I call the number. "Hey, my name is Tim Grutzius, and I am a firefighter with the Alsip Fire Department. I am interested in knowing more about what you have to offer. Unfortunately, I can't make it to your workshop tomorrow."

Sarah, a clinical counsellor on the other end of the line, tells me more about the workshop. Somehow, the trauma of a previous call enters the conversation, and despite my best efforts to repress it, I talk. Sarah then suggests, "We are offering a first responder's workshop at a later date. Would you like to tell your story there? We also are forming a group called Illinois Firefighter Peer Support. You should apply and attend the three-day training to become a peer supporter."

"I would love to," I find myself saying.

I sit down to write out the fifteen-minute presentation I will be giving at the first workshop. It is about a work-related incident that happened years ago. I am sure I am over it.

But I am wrong, so very wrong. When I recall the night, the call, the explosion, the charred, burned body of a man who had drowned himself in gasoline before lighting the match, the smell and taste of deployed fire extinguishers that were too little, too late, the death by suicide, the realization that the body was that of my colleague, my *friend*, a fellow firefighter—all the old feelings bubble up, unexpectedly resurfacing.

I find myself in front of the audience, ready to share my story. I start to utter the first sentence, and I break down in tears.

What is the matter with you, Tim? You know this story. You are over it.

I stumble through the words, surviving the longest fifteen minutes of my life.

As I walk out, Sarah pulls me aside. "You might want to prepare yourself for the three-day training workshop. It might be tough."

I am confident. "Anything after that speech will be easy."

Of course, I am wrong.

It is the second day of the workshop when Sarah explains all the symptoms of post-traumatic stress disorder. I see myself in everything she says.

"I have a problem," I mouth.

It's hard to fight a fire you simply cannot see. But I can see it now.

I have a problem. It is raging inside, silently consuming and burning me, and it has a name. It is not just impatience learned from childhood or annoyance at bad drivers. It is PTSD. I have experienced trauma—trauma in my childhood, trauma in my career, trauma in my life—and I need to process it. I need to live an examined life. I am not an idiot or a bad person like I so often tell myself. I am sick, and I am ready to start a healing journey. I want to learn how to be a better colleague, husband, friend. I want to feel peace.

I decide to reach out for help, for counselling, for support. I want to quell and control the fire that is PTSD. I want to be a different type of firefighter. It is time to rescue myself; to be a better and happier me; to work toward a balanced life in mind, body, and spirit.

I discover an arsenal of modalities to help me fight my internal fire—regular exercise, healthy eating, meditation, yoga, chiropractic care, massage therapy, and Reiki treatments help me stay grounded.

I find myself on the same highway when an inconsiderate driver cuts me off. I do not react. I simply go with the flow.

Judy smiles. She touches my shoulder, not with a jab, but with gratitude. "I am so glad you only drive big red vehicles with lights and sirens at work now."

I have tears in my eyes because I know that I could never have made it this far without her enduring and selfless love.

Daphne Rose Kingma once wrote, "Holding on is believing that there's only a past; letting go is knowing that there's a future."

Currently a lieutenant, Tim Grutzius is a twenty-four-year veteran of the Alsip Fire Department. Tim has been married to his best friend and wife, Judy, a third-grade teacher, for twenty-two years. He owns a business called Cent' Anni Life where he seeks to work with whomever requests his services. His particular focus is on those who are under a great deal of stress like first responders, military veterans, educators, or anyone with whom his story resonates. For more information, please visit centannilife.com.

CAMPING

Diane McKay

"WHERE WOULD YOU LIKE TO go camping?" my husband, Alan, asks.

Subtle concern inches up into my core. "Are you sure you want to try camping?"

"Why wouldn't I?"

My radar fires off in all directions.

"Well, you haven't been camping before."

"Yes, I have."

"Where?" I challenge.

"I've been to holiday camps back in England," he announces.

"Hardly the same as camping in a tent . . . here . . . in Canada. Not quite the same as the wilds of Southwest London."

My concern warrants consideration, I believe, as Alan is always too hot, too cold, too uncomfortable, too tired, too anxious, too bored, too hungry, too, too, too, too . . . Once a professional soccer player, his arthritis is more prevalent than a non-descript Nickelback song: same chords, different title. He aches—his back, his knee, his elbow. They all fire off, exasperated, if ever he encounters an uncomfortable bed. How on earth could he manage to sleep in a tent? On the ground? In the woods?

He picks up on my concern, barraging me with roughneck, backwoods, tough-guy questions about Ontario's provincial parks:

How hot are the showers? Are there any bears? Is there running water? And the clincher, how do you lock your tent at night?

This does not bolster my confidence. In fact, I remember early on in our relationship when he told me a story about when he first moved to Canada. He was in some rural parts, and he was introduced to a real-life outhouse. After experiencing this amazing invention for the first time, he spent a half hour looking for the "chain" as he called it. He spent thirty minutes trying to figure out how to flush the toilet—in an outhouse—and he wants to go camping?

However, my father had sold his cottage the year before, we were broke, and I really wanted to get away for a few days.

"I've always wanted to go to Bon Echo," I venture.

Thanks to the Internet and a credit card that has just enough room on it, we sign up for four nights.

Lately, Alan's mental health has been declining. Obsessively feasting on the negativity often found on social media, his depression gained weight, swelling to almost obese proportions. I hope this trip will go well. I am a seasoned camper, but I wonder how he will handle the new experience. I make him watch numerous YouTube videos on how to set up air mattresses and how to stay warm at night. This is one "too" I don't wish to deal with.

We arrive at Bon Echo Provincial Park right after a thunder storm. Finding our little plot, we unload all the gear. There is a lot of it, and things are disorganized. He becomes flustered, overwhelmed, and starts to shut down. With Alan, regrouping, although eventual, is reluctant. My agitation increases, and I wonder if four nights was too optimistic. His mood improves, however, as we create order, setting up camp. With the tiny three-man tent erected, he asks, "Where's the lid?"

Pause. "Ummm, you mean the fly?"

"Yeah, that and all."

"Over here."

We drape the protective sheet over the tent, first inside out, then we get it right.

"I have to go to the bathroom," he announces.

"Okay, don't be too long. It is almost dusk."

I start to pump up the air mattresses. One done. Then two. I set up the camp stove. I share some pistachios with neighbouring chipmunks. Where is he? He has been gone a long time. Just as I am about to find a park ranger to send out a search party, Alan comes sauntering back into the campsite.

"Where were you?"

"I went to the bathroom."

"It took you that long?"

"Well, there was a bit of a problem. The bathrooms were all locked. The electricity went out with the storm, and everything was shut," he begins his story.

"So what did you do?" I regret it as soon as the words leave my mouth.

"I went in the woods."

"You *what*?"

"I had to go. I couldn't wait. So I found a spot in the woods, but . . ."

Uh oh, is all I can think.

"When I was finished, I started to stand up, and there was this woman on a bike coming down the pathway. I was back farther in the woods but not too far from where the path makes a sharp turn. We were staring right at each other, face to face, right before she had to turn on the path."

"What did you do?"

"I said 'hi' and lowered myself back down again."

I am utterly mortified. Is this a sign of things to come?

Then he says, "I love it here. I don't care if I have to sleep on the ground or go to the bathroom in the woods. You have to see this."

"What is it?" I ask.

He doesn't answer. Instead he grabs my hand and we rush off.

On the pathway, he points out the spot. "This is where I . . ."

I interrupt. "You didn't bring me here to show me *that*, surely?"

"What does Shirley have to do with anything?" Damn British humour.

"No," he laughs.

We continue on and follow a bend in the path that opens up to the Mazinaw Rock, a cliff face jutting out from the lake; the dusk sun burnishes the spectacular sight with brilliant yellows and golds, creating a whole new version of sepia, one I have never experienced before.

We are silent. In that pivotal moment, I actually can't speak. Sight beyond words. Beauty beyond amplification. Spirit beyond form. We are awestruck, like the many Indigenous people who traversed this waterway before us, leaving their legacy of the two hundred and sixty pictographs that are as solid as the rock face they are marked upon.

Eventually we go back to our campsite. We burn supper, a raccoon makes off with a twenty-dollar Costco-sized bag of pistachios, our campsite is sandwiched between flatulent neighbours to the right and snorers to the left, we trip while trying to drag our fifty-year-plus bodies into the hobbit-sized tent door, we sleep on air mattresses. On the ground. In a tent . . . and we love it. Most importantly, *Alan* loves it!

It is healing. Alan is up early. He hikes. He learns how to start the camp stove. He loves to do the dishes in a plastic bucket. He falls into the lake while trying to get into a kayak (and laughs). He learns where the water pump is and that yes, indeed, the showers have hot water. You don't even need to lock your tent! But mostly, he disconnects. Our campsite does not have power, and that is powerful.

The only screen time we experience is the stars in the night sky; the only mobiles we have are our feet; the only ones tweeting are birds; the only trolls are raccoons; and the only thing "insta" is our over-priced freeze-dried meals we bought from the camping specialty store.

Turns out my trepidation is unfounded. Beauty triumphs vile, healing beats injury, and love conquers fear. It is the best trip ever—for both of us. Now, when life gets a little too much and the information highway attempts to steal our joy, we remember the good echo of ourselves we experienced camping and remember that sometimes the best way to connect is to disconnect.

Diane McKay is a mother and a wife. Since this experience, she has been camping with Alan numerous times. Diane loves running, knitting, and basically anything humorous.

GINGERBREAD MEN

Kate Lyon Osher

THE FIRST HOLIDAY SEASON SINCE Greg died by suicide rolls around, and I want nothing to do with it. I am staying with my parents, and my mom is like me. She goes all out for Christmas (I wonder where I get it from). But this year, I dread the decorations, the tree, the lights, the joy. I have no fa-la-la-la-la spirit in me. I look more like the Grinch or Scrooge, and I would happily move into a dark cave and hibernate until the fifteenth of January if it were an option.

For much of my relationship with my late husband, Greg, we lived in different states. I was in California finishing up college and grad school, and he was in Colorado furthering his tech-industry career. We did our best to see each other monthly and always during the holidays. He would come out for Thanksgiving, or in the years he was with his family, I would head out shortly thereafter. If we weren't together for Christmas, we were always together from December twenty-sixth through the New Year. The way we often rang in the start of the holiday season was with my favourite gingerbread ice cream sandwiches. They came out every Thanksgiving to all the chain grocery stores and stayed through the end of January.

Oftentimes, I stocked up so my stash would last at least through Valentine's Day.

I don't remember who made them, and they were probably mostly made of things we couldn't pronounce, but they were soft gingerbread cookies sandwiched together with vanilla ice cream. And they were damn delicious. I ate them during finals; I ate them writing papers; I ate them whenever I wanted to feel like I was eating Christmas.

If Greg was in California, they were in my freezer. If I was in Colorado, they were in Greg's freezer. No matter what was happening in life, those gingerbread men made everything better. They were, in many ways, a holiday glue. When things were amazing and we couldn't love each other any better, we had those treats. When things were not so great and we did things that hurt each other, or we made choices that caused pain to the other, those treats gave us common ground again. When things were bad, they were a sugary-sweet peace pipe that meant all was forgiven.

So when my mom starts to get rolling on the house transformation on the first of December, I boogie to the local Ralph's to see if I can eat my feelings. I know that a gingerbread man ice cream sandwich (or six, or twelve, or the entire stock) will help me regulate the knots in my stomach.

When I get to the frozen novelty aisle where they have been stocked for as long as I can remember and I see none, I know there has to be a mistake. Perhaps they are being spotlighted in an end-of-aisle display. No dice. I go back to the frozen section and see a clerk stocking shelves.

I ask her, "Where are the gingerbread men?"

She turns to me with a blank look. "I have no idea."

Wondering how she has ever made it this far in life in the frozen section without knowing about them, I inquire, "Can you ask the store manager?"

"Sure," she answers and walks toward the back of the store. She returns a minute later. "The store manager says we aren't getting any more."

I am incredulous. This can't be true. "You are kidding. Really? Can you please ask the store manager to come to the aisle?"

I show the manager where the gingerbread ice cream men had been displayed every end of November to the end of January since I could remember, and I ask, "Why aren't they there?"

The manager then tells me what is the absolute last thing I need to hear. "They aren't making the gingerbread ice cream treats anymore. We won't be getting any. Ever."

And, with this, I feel the wind being knocked out of me. I am freezing—more freezing than you should be after standing in the frozen foods section for ten minutes. Then, out of the depth of my being, it starts. The waterworks. The sobbing. The uncontrollable babble of someone in grief. I drop to my knees while the clerk and manager just look at each other, and then the manager pulls out his walkie-talkie.

Other customers are surrounding me. Then a security guard. All of this at the grocery store in my hometown where I have been shopping with my mom since pretty much birth. After what seems like an hour of me blathering on about gingerbread men, the security guard asks, "Do you think you might be able to walk outside?"

"No," I answer.

"Can we call someone?" the manager chimes in.

I give them my parents' home number.

A few minutes later, my dear father comes in, looking concerned and sad, and sits down beside me, explaining to the lookie-loos and the store personnel, "She has suffered a pretty significant loss, and the holidays are going to be hard. Please just give us a minute, and we will be on our way."

It doesn't take much to realize this isn't really about gingerbread men ice cream sandwiches (but hell if I won't miss them every year). It is about love and loss and the finality that comes with knowing the life you had isn't the life you have anymore. It is grief. It is having to look at the past—the good, the bad, and the ugly—and knowing I have to deal with all of it if I want any chance at any sort of future.

It is coming to terms with the fact that I have to find a way to make a new path for myself out of the unfamiliar, that Greg and the gingerbread men ice cream sandwiches aren't coming back, and I have to come to terms with that.

I am surprised I don't make it into the DAILY CRIME section of the local paper. I still enjoy gingerbread men ice cream sandwiches, just in a different way. I bake my own gingerbread men and slather some vanilla bean ice cream in between. Sometimes I take the store-bought gingerbread cookies and do the same thing. And they taste pretty darn good. Of course, it's not the same as the original, but I learn it doesn't have to be. It's different, but in a good way. The memory of the old treat remains, but it isn't painful anymore. It doesn't render me a sobbing mess in the middle of a grocery store with security on my heels.

It's the same with my life. I've had to make adjustments in the years since Greg has been gone. I have had to find a new path. It doesn't mean I don't remember Greg. It doesn't mean I don't miss him. The difference between then and now is that I can look back and not be consumed with the gut-wrenching sadness I had for so long. I have let love in again—and it's made me whole.

In looking for some new gingerbread men ice cream sandwiches, I took some turns that led me to the wonderful life I currently have, with love and laughter and a husband who prefers brownies over gingerbread, and little boys who love gingerbread cookies just as much as their mama does. And when one of my sons cries when he realizes he just bit off and ate the head of his beloved gingerbread pal, I can hug him and kiss him and giggle at the power of DNA.

Kate Lyon Osher is a wife, a mom, a sister, a daughter, an aunt, and a friend who became a survivor of suicide loss in 2002. She is an attorney who lives in California. She writes, speaks, and does all she can to remove the stigma associated with discussing mental health. You can follow her blog at mamalawmadingdong.com.

BRENT RETURNS

L.A. Hill

MY HUSBAND IS A PILOT. He is a good man. Sometimes I feel he is too good, or so I keep telling myself. Feeling secure and cared for without worry is something I am not used to. Peace and normalcy can make me feel uncomfortable while I spend my time anxiously awaiting the next penny to drop.

It is a beautiful afternoon, and I am preparing dinner and eagerly anticipating my husband's arrival after several days on the road. Wine—an hour earlier I opened a bottle. By the time he arrives, I have nearly finished it, and all my buried insecurities rise to the surface. He enters the house. I am in the kitchen and do not hear his voice calling. I walk to the hallway to see him at the door. He is quiet and appears to momentarily avoid eye contact, not his usual effusive self.

All my senses heighten, a plethora of negative scenarios ruminating uncontrollably in my head. Of course he is probably just tired from several days of work, battling the traffic as he drove up from the city, and simply happy to be home. But I do not allow any of *those* possibilities to take up residence in my head.

I blow it *again*. My self-sabotaging, accusatory body of pain surfaces, causing chaos in my life. We erupt into a thirty-minute shouting match of accusations, indignation, and hurtful words, followed by an exit out the same door that my husband entered a mere half-hour before. He drives away.

Brent is gone. I am left alone. I sob.

When I was six years old, my family drove across the country from Kamloops, British Columbia, to London, Ontario, for a family reunion, my first true adventure. I was taken out of school for the trip, and my parents weren't their usual argumentative selves. I experienced staying in a hotel, getting carsick and throwing up over the Rocky Mountains, and losing a tooth, only to learn that the Tooth Fairy could find me even if I was sleeping in a hotel. I loved this trip, too, because my dad was relaxed, and I really enjoyed spending time with him.

The first day after arriving in London, my dad and uncle insisted on going out.

"Can I come?" I begged.

"No, Lynn-Anne, not this time. We will do something together tomorrow," my dad placated me.

I spent the day in town, endlessly wandering stores with my mother and grandmother instead.

Later that evening in my grandmother's guest room, I remember standing up on the bed and looking out the window at the lights of the city. It was raining, and I was still upset my father had left without me . . . until I wasn't.

Something inside me realized he wasn't coming back . . . *ever*. I felt strangely calm, anger draining from my body.

Doorbell. Police officers. Accident.

He was gone. I was left.

After cleaning up the kitchen, I check a tracking app on my cellphone that we use for our child's safety to see if I can locate

Brent. Forty minutes up north . . . where is he going? I'm scared. What if he doesn't return? I begin negotiating with the universe and chant gratitude for my husband's love and understanding.

After my father's funeral, I remember my grandmother offered to take me back with her to St. John's, Newfoundland, for what I understood to be a visit.

"It will be the best for everybody," she said.

I went. At first it was nice. But seasons came and went, and I enrolled in school. I heard from my mother, who lived in Montreal, less and less. I wondered why. My mother always had a new explanation, or excuse, as to why I couldn't move back—new boyfriend, just moved in with someone. Even when I did go visit, I was treated more like a guest than a daughter. On one visit, she arrived drunk at the airport to pick me up, and I was given a mattress on the floor in the rec room to serve as my bedroom.

Mom was gone. I was left.

I want to call Brent but hesitate. I urge the telephone to ring— and it does. Scared, I don't answer it the first time. He calls again and I pick up. "I'm sorry . . . please come home."

"I am angry and I'm hurt. I am also tired of arguing with you," he explains.

We continue to talk.

Before my first son's birth, I was with his dad for six years. It was idyllic. I was a Sunday School teacher and he was a deacon. I became pregnant right before he lost his job. He moved to Toronto from Montreal, promising to visit. He did visit . . . he just didn't visit *me*.

He was gone. I was left.

I can see on the cellphone app that my husband is no longer driving away from me. He is heading toward home, *toward me*.

"We should talk to a counsellor," he suggests. My heart begins to pound and I say, "I want to work it out on our own without anyone else's involvement."

"Beautiful," he responds, "we need to get some help. You've experienced traumatic abandonment, and I can't handle bearing the brunt of what others have done to you."

My anxious mind warns that counselling will result in judgment and loss of control over my marriage; however, I know my husband is right.

"I know. Yes, it's a good idea," I say weakly, trying to silence the desperate voice inside.

"Love you."

"Love you, too."

I am left to consider our discourse, my life, our love, our commitment. Contemplation steals my thoughts until I look down at my phone and see on the app that Brent's car is back at our house.

Brent is home. So am I.

As we embrace, I realize that I don't need to weigh every relationship on the scales of my past experiences. Constantly testing to see if my bliss is just a precursor to abandonment isn't serving me . . . or Brent for that matter.

"I'm glad you returned," I say.

"So am I," he answers.

L.A. Hill, entrepreneur, sailor, wannabe jetsetter, lifelong pursuer of positivity, and first-time writer, avidly produces and promotes initiatives to end the stigma of mental illness. To learn more about what L.A. is up to, visit Eventsbylabarrie on Facebook.

CALLING FOR ME

Zoey Raffay

I CLENCH THE KNIFE HANDLE until my knuckles turn white as I glance down at the long, sharp blade. I admire it, twisting it in my hand. It reflects and shines the moonlight onto my bedroom wall. *This knife is the answer to my pain*, I think and inwardly chuckle at the irony. And I know that no one will understand. I need to die—it's not a want at this point; it's an agonizing need. My mental pain is too great. Like the musty leaves I will hide this knife under when I am through with carving out my pain, I have been tossed aside, too—by happiness. I promise that I have begged on my knees to feel joy, but I have never found it . . . or maybe it has never found me. I have to sneak out of the house now. This isn't going to be easy with my family downstairs, but I've realized that my dead body belongs in the woods. I will be standing there soon, knife in my hand and a clear plan to die.

You don't understand, Charlie. I know you're my best friend, but you still don't understand. I can't take it anymore, I text with my fingers shaking in anger. *No one understands my pain*, I think to myself as I continue: My parents are constantly fighting, I never get to see my boyfriend or go out with friends, so why do I even bother being alive?

You have so much to live for, Charlie replies, seemingly unaffected, or so I think.

Give me one thing! I reply. *Go for it*, I think. Whatever she comes up with will be meaningless to me. She doesn't understand depression—she just doesn't!

You have your future. Think about how your parents would react when they see your lifeless body. Imagine how your siblings, friends, and even teachers would feel if you decide to take your life.

Sigh. I don't think anyone would miss me. I am worthless, and I don't do any good for anyone. I text with what energy I have left to explain myself:

I can't take how I feel inside anymore. I need to just die.

I put the phone down. I'm done with explaining this to anyone. I have already said goodbye to my little brothers and given them a massive hug. It will be quick—death is now around the corner for me. I won't see my sixteenth birthday, and I definitely don't care.

I write a note to leave behind.

To Whoever finds this note,

I am sorry I disappointed you. I am sorry that I caused tears to come to your eyes, but what you have to understand is that I couldn't take what was going on in my head anymore. I am getting bullied at school, my grades are dropping, and I feel like the whole school, including the teachers, hate me. I'm tired of people judging me. I can't stand the way I think about myself. It's all gotten to be too much for me. I just can't do it anymore. I've tried to hold on for as long as I could, but eventually my hand let go of the rope and I fell.

Zach, I'm sorry, buddy. I know you don't understand right now, but I know when you're older you will. Do something big with your life, and don't let anyone stand in your way of doing what you want. You are one of the best little brothers ever. Don't ever change from being the positive loving person you are. I love you, buddy, and don't ever forget that.

Eli, I am sorry, bud-bud, for hurting you. I didn't want to, but I had no choice. You are a very intelligent little boy. Continue doing what you love and take care of Zach for me. I love you, E. Always remember that.

Mya, hey I know that I hurt you even though you may not be showing it. I know I did. I am sorry for everything—for the fights I picked with you, for always being a bully to you; it wasn't fair and I apologize deeply. Keep working out and playing hockey. I am one hundred percent positive that, if you keep working toward your goal of becoming an Olympic hockey player, you will succeed. Know that I'll be looking down and cheering you on.

Mom and Dad, you guys have been amazing parents. I couldn't have asked for better ones. You did everything in your power for us, even if money was tight. You guys are incredible. I don't know how you raised four kids, but you guys did a great job of it. I love you so much more than words could ever describe. I just couldn't take the voices and the negative cloud that was hovering above my head any longer, and I apologize. I know that this will be a barrier for you to overcome, but I'm sure you'll get over it. I'm not worth much anyway.

As for everyone else, I don't want anyone coming to my grave and telling me how much you guys love me and how you will miss me. Don't grieve over me. All I want you to do is look up at the sky and say goodbye.

I'm sorry . . . goodbye.

Suddenly, I hear a siren in the distance. No big deal. Then it gets closer . . . and closer. *NO!* I scream in my mind. I run to my phone and find what I am dreading I would find—another text from Charlie.

I'm calling 9-1-1. I'm sorry. I'm worried about you.

I fall to my knees, the knife bouncing onto the carpet as I release it from my grasp.

Nooo! She actually has called the cops on me? How could she do this to me? I hate her so much!

I quickly shove the knife into my closet while I hear my mom answer the front door. "Hello, ma'am. We were called to check on your daughter Zoey. We have been informed by a friend that she may be considering harming herself." That's when my world stops. I have nowhere to hide. I can't run from my pain anymore. Now my mom knows I'm suicidal.

The ambulance ride is embarrassing. I hate Charlie so much right now. How are these paramedics actually going to help me? Yeah, sure, they are nice, but what do they know about depression? Thankfully my mom sits in the front of the ambulance while one of the paramedics talks to me in the back.

"Were you wanting to hurt yourself, Zoey?"

What should I say? This is so pointless. She won't understand. "Yes." Fine, I'll just be honest.

"Do you have a plan?" the paramedic asks.

"Yes." She looks at me as if that's not enough of an answer. "I'm going to take pills, and if that doesn't work, I'm going to cut myself."

Are you happy now, Miss Paramedic?

"I'm sorry to hear that," she says.

"No one understands," I say as tears well up in my eyes.

"I do," she replies.

What? Is this a joke? "What do you mean?" I ask.

"I have depression. I take medications for it. I have also wanted to kill myself before."

"Are you serious?" I ask, wiping my tears away.

"I wouldn't lie to you, Zoey. I have had the same day that you are having today. My friend also called 9-1-1 for me."

"*For* you? You mean *on* you," I say, still frustrated with Charlie.

"Well, at first I felt that way, too," she says while passing me a tissue. "But I see it differently now. Maybe you will, too, one day. My friend saved my life. Yes, I didn't want to be saved at first, but I am happy now that I have gotten the help I needed to be alive."

Help? I guess I never thought of it as "help" before.

Now, a year later, I kick the leaves as I walk along the wooded path. Their musty smell wafts up toward my nose—the smell that I would have buried my knife in had I taken my life that day. A robin chirps in a nearby tree, and I catch myself smiling at it. Life is . . . good. I see a counsellor for my depression now, and I am on medications that seem to help me a lot. Charlie and I aren't the best of friends, but I can say this: She saved my life that day. She called 9-1-1 *for* me. I didn't see it that way at first, but it's hard to see things clearly in the dark. It's hard to see anything when the only light you see is the moonlight reflecting off a blade while you wait to take your last breath. Thank you, Charlie, for helping me to see that there is also sunlight.

Zoey Raffay is a seventeen-year-old from Ontario. She loves to run, read, shop, and spend time with her family. She has two brothers and a sister whom she loves dearly.

DILLON

Julie Jolicoeur

"I CAN'T HAVE THAT DOG on the plane," I hear the well-dressed woman sitting a few rows up and across from me say. "I'm afraid of him."

Dillon, a placid golden retriever, lies by my feet. I feel my pulse quicken. We have just taken off.

"I am sorry, Ma'am. That is a service dog; there is nothing I can do," the attendant explains.

"I want him off the plane. I don't want to fly with him," she counters.

I feel anxiety creeping up. What if I am asked to get off the plane? We have just left Newark, a busy airport at best, a nightmare for me to navigate at worst. What if I can't get home?

The flight attendant continues to attempt to placate the disgruntled passenger. "I am sorry. He has all his papers. There is nothing we can do. You can, however, move back to the middle of the plane where there are some empty seats if you would like to sit farther away."

"No, I don't want to move. This is *my* seat."

"I simply cannot help you." The flight attendant ends the conversation.

My friends and I are returning back to Ottawa from a geocaching trip in Cincinnati. For some, this may seem like a simple trip—a vacation with friends. However, leaving my kids and husband behind for such an adventure is a big deal when, for almost eight years, leaving the confines of my house was close to impossible.

I feel the familiar symptoms of a panic attack setting in. My cortisol levels rise and so does Dillon—as he is trained to do. He puts his paws on my lap so that I engage in petting him, grounding me, bringing me back to the present.

The woman's attitude has unnerved me, and my stress does not dissipate. Dillon continues to climb, one leg, then the other, into my lap, paws on either shoulder, pinning me to my seat, the pressure calming me.

"Are you okay?" my friend Steve, who is sitting a few rows back, asks.

I am pinned so tightly I cannot turn to answer.

Dillon is not moving and neither am I for the entire hour and twenty-minute flight.

I used to volunteer, raising seeing-eye dogs. Somehow, it was okay to help those with physical disabilities; however, I didn't want my private battle with mental illness to become a public one by having a service dog. I felt like it would invade my privacy, like I had a stamp on my forehead that said, I HAVE A MENTAL ILLNESS.

But eventually, being a prisoner in my own house was less appealing than letting the world know my condition, so I applied for a service dog, resulting in Dillon.

We land and thankfully deplane. I am tired, drained, and depleted from the trip. I see a man in the airport with a cellphone about to snap a shot of Dillon and me. I know that Dillon is adorable and is a beautiful dog, but I am simply not in the mood. I interrupt his process: "Please don't take a picture of me." I wonder, *Would he take a picture of someone in a wheelchair? Probably not.*

He puts his phone away.

A wheelchair is a medical device and in a way so is Dillon. Most people have never thought of it like that, though. Sometimes I don't like all the questions; sometimes I am just in a hurry and want to get the milk and run out of the store without someone asking me why I have a service dog—or what his name is; and sometimes . . . I just want to blend in. There are times I want to be invisible and wear the mask of normalcy, which is nearly impossible with a service dog.

I realize that just like there are side effects for many drug therapies such as weight gain, dry mouth, or headaches, my therapy—Dillon—has a major side effect, too: lack of privacy. Unlike suffering from heart disease or diabetes that may not be apparent at first glance, my condition is announced to those around me simply by his presence. When considering any medical intervention, the risks versus benefits are always weighed. And although I know it is a trade-off, it is the right one for me.

I go to the store now. I take walks, run errands, travel. In fact, I even leave my husband and kids at home and fly off to Cincinnati with friends to geocache. That can almost be classified as a miracle.

Home, I look at my beautiful dog. Dillon lies calmly at my feet, his breathing steady and calming.

"Dillon," I say as I stroke his soft, golden fur. "Life is so much better with you in it. In a way, you have allowed me to live again. Thank you."

I kiss the top of his big head, turn out the light, and go to bed. Tomorrow I will wake up and will be able to do the things I want to, the things I never used to, the things some people take for granted. Even though there can be minor annoyances like disgruntled plane passengers or curious people with cameras, I truly can't imagine life without a service dog now. When it comes to Dillon, the pros outweigh the cons by unfathomable lengths. And for this, I am truly grateful.

Julie Jolicoeur is a proud mother of two daughters, a wife of a paramedic, and a former primary-care paramedic with the City of Ottawa. She was diagnosed with post-traumatic stress disorder in 2005 and has been on the road to recovery ever since.

SUNBURN

Matthew Heneghan

IN THE WANING DAYS OF winter, the sun begins to clasp itself to the sky above for a little longer each day, reminding us of an impending summer. I hate the summer. I hate the heat. I hate the sun and the sun hates me. I am aware that it is impossible for the sun to actually harbour ill will for me, but it certainly feels as though it does. Allow me to elaborate.

I hate the sun because I have been burned by it. Not in the superficial vexation of reddened skin and postliminary flakes, not at all; something else entirely . . .

I can recall the first reason I hate the sun. I remember the day, or rather, the sequential group of days, in May. I remember being a young, fresh-faced soldier in the Canadian army. I was at the garrison, sitting in the back of a dust-coated military ambulance, taking inventory of expired and damaged supplies. The sun was overhead and beat down in a relentless and punitive manner. A cascading beam of light broke its way through a petite-sized hole in the top corner of the back of the ambulance, searing a permanent scar into my memory. Dust and particles alike danced in defiance of gravity through the laser-like pillar of light. The term "sweltering" does not accurately depict the oven-like bake that we were sitting in.

As a private and I rummaged through med bags and cabinets, discarding expired supplies, a deep baritone voice broke in from behind us. We spun around to meet whatever commands awaited us from our sergeant, a kind but disciplined man. "Relax. Take a seat."

He stood at the back of the ambulance with squinted gaze beneath the boasting sun. What followed was a painful reminder of the chosen profession that we were in—he spoke with unrehearsed empathy. "A man is dead."

I sat and listened intently to each of his spoken words. My ears perked with intrigue while my eyes struggled to remain unencumbered of tears. It was not simply a man who had died, it was a fellow medic, a friend, a brother. The sun watched Corporal Michael Starker die that day, and now it peered through the back canopy of an aging ambulance and watched as a little piece of me did as well. It watched mercilessly and apathetically as I fought against every instinct to break and wail like a wounded civilian.

"Take the time you need, pull yourself together, and then come inside. I will break the news to the unit post-lunch."

"Yes, Sergeant."

The sergeant walked away briskly, and I remained manacled to the bench seat in the back of the ambulance. The private tried to speak to me, but I shrugged off his attempts. Filled with anger and grief, I barked, "Shut up!"

The sun followed me for the next few days. It followed me home and then to the bar. It rose the next morning, slapping me and my hangover in the face. It tailed me to the funeral hall in Calgary, and it continued to mock me from above when I stood graveside, watching as my friend was lowered into the earth.

The heat from the sun permeated our pristinely pressed green uniforms. It laughed as sweat greeted tears and melted into the collars of our shirts. It just hung above as if perched on a throne, watching as peons grieved and mourned the loss of a man. The sun was bright, but the birds were silent. Only heat could be felt, and only the bereft clatter of rifle rounds overhead could be heard.

During those gut-wrenching days in May, I hated the sun. And every year when I revisit days in May, I hate it all over again.

The sun was also bright and sinister two years prior when my twenty-three-year-old friend Boomer was killed by a suicide bomber. Then there was July, a bright day in July, when I got the call. "Henny, it's Colin . . . Colin is dead. I'm really sorry, man."

Another friend. Another medic. Another loss. Another sunny day.

And the sun continued to shine in November. The November when my phone woke me while I was burdened by my everyday adversarial hangover, coming to life with a ring that was shot from a cannon.

I clasped the phone within my hand and pressed it against my cheek. I managed a cordial "hello."

I lay motionless and listened to the voice on the other end of the line, the voice of my brother, stammering and piercing through the perforated holes of my speaker. His grief-stricken words were utterances that I will never forget: "Matt, Mom's dead."

On an irritatingly sunny day at the start of November, my mother died by way of suicide.

This heart-shattering day was a disgustingly beautiful one outside. The sun loomed high throughout the vastness of space and beamed down brightly with a limitless roar—a direct contrast to how I was feeling.

I painfully undertook the task of reading my mother's suicide note. I did so beneath the casting light of a burning sun. Every word, every line, and the sun just skulked and sneered overhead.

The sun accompanies most people while on vacation. For me however, all the sun brings to me is heartache and pain with overwhelming loss.

Sun: one, two, three, four . . .

Matt: zero

Today, the sun rises, and so do I. I go outside and notice something new, foreign, but almost comforting—warmth. In fact, the sun and I feel amicable. I guess, through the help of therapy and introspective objectivity, I have come to realize that the sun is neither sinister nor compassionate. The sun is merely the sun. It is what it is. It does not judge or antagonize. It simply just exists.

If I can accept something I used to detest and loathe, perhaps I can do the same with the demons of post-traumatic stress disorder. Maybe I can forgive myself and let go of the things that I have seen and done when working as a paramedic. In time, I will learn to forgive myself for being unable to save my own mother.

The sun brings light to new days. And that is what I am learning to focus on—new days. Brighter days. Seeking light instead of living in the dark. I wake up each day even when I don't want to. I get out of bed in spite of my wounded mind telling me not to. And I step out of my home into an awaiting sun and continue to feel its warmth even though I once felt its unmistakable burn. I am healing because I. Am. Living.

Am I sick? Yes. Wounded? Yes. But I am not weak. And as sure as the sun continues to rise, so will hope.

Matthew Heneghan is thirty-five years old, and his story is one that begins with his decision to serve his country as a medic in the Canadian Armed Forces. He served six years and was honourably discharged in 2008. Upon his release, he became a paramedic for the city of Edmonton, where he worked for almost seven years. Matthew relocated to Toronto, Ontario, in 2014, and started a journey of self discovery. He was diagnosed with post-traumatic stress disorder in 2017. Since then, he has been in therapy and continues to heal, learn, and grow. Read more of Matthew's musings at amedicsmind.com.

KEEP RIDING

Heidi Allen

I GO TO VISIT MY younger sister. We haven't always been close, but over the last few years, things have really improved. Though we live in two different cities an hour and a half apart, we're closer than we've ever been.

We don't see each other often, but we call or text almost every day. Sometimes both.

I knock on the door. "So good to see you." We hug.

I go inside, and it isn't long until we reminisce about our childhood and chat about our everyday lives. It feels great to be as connected as we are.

Today our talk centres on some health issues my sister's been going through. She's struggling with a physical illness, and it is affecting her mental health—emotionally struggling with the question of when things are going to get better.

We've all had times like these. I've had many throughout my lifetime—times where I couldn't see the light at the end of the tunnel. Instead I could only see the darkness I had to feel my way through. I could sympathize.

I desperately want to give her some hope that eventually her troubles would be over. I share this story with her.

Last summer, my husband, Mike, and I decided to go for an adventure on his motorcycle. We rode up to Ottawa to reconnect with some old friends over a long weekend. The ride was amazing, and so was the rest of the weekend.

Sadly, the fun came to an end when it was time to head home. Mike checked the weather and broke the bad news to me: It was supposed to rain for the entire day.

I was a little nervous, but we agreed there was no way that was going to stop us. We donned our rain gear, hopped on the Harley, and started the journey home.

We didn't feel a drop of rain for the first thirty minutes but could see dark storm clouds brewing in the distance. "How you doing back there?" Mike asked, his voice coming through the speaker in my helmet.

"I'm good, but those clouds look scary," I responded.

"We're heading into some bad weather, but hopefully it won't be for too long."

Within ten minutes, we hit the rain. Actually, the rain hit us. Not a drizzle, not a playful shower, but a fierce, torrential downpour. As the rain fell, so did the temperature. I tightened my arms around Mike.

"We're only about twenty minutes to the first rest stop," he yelled. "Are you okay back there?"

"I'm okay," I said, beginning to feel a little unsure.

The rain beat down on my helmet and bike suit, the sound of it roaring all around me. I couldn't believe how loud it was, giving the motorcycle's engine a run for its money.

When we arrived at the first rest stop, we grabbed a coffee and sat by the window. I stared out at the parking lot and watched Mike's motorcycle get assaulted by the rain. I held my coffee with both hands and savoured its warmth on my skin.

"I've looked at the weather, and it doesn't look like the rain is going to let up. Are you good to keep going?" Mike asked, looking up from his phone.

"How far is it to the next stop?"

"It's only eighty-six kilometres and under an hour." He looked out at his bike and then back at me. "We can do it!" he started chanting.

I smiled at him. Of course we could do it.

"Let's do it!"

Minutes into the next leg of our journey, my confidence started to waver. I felt incredibly cold and knew I had many hours of this misery before we got home.

I just wanted to be home—warm, dry, and safe.

That's when a little voice in my head, my inner Heidi, said, "You can do this! All you have to do is focus on getting to the next rest stop. Don't think about how far home is. Only concentrate on the next eighty-six kilometres."

So, for the next eighty-six kilometres, I clung to this thought as tightly as I clung to Mike. The distance home didn't seem quite so scary anymore. I couldn't believe it. I'd given myself a pep talk, and it actually seemed to be working.

A very short time later, we were sitting in the next rest stop. My rain gear was wet and I couldn't seem to get warm, but I felt quite proud of myself.

Twenty minutes later, we were back on the bike. Before we took off, I asked Mike how far it was to the next stop.

Mike set the odometer. "We only have eighty-seven kilometres to go."

Eighty-seven? That was nothing.

"I can do this," I muttered to myself.

By the time we got to the next pit stop, my clothes were soaked through, my teeth chattered, and the rain felt like a barrage of small rocks pummelling my skin. But sitting there with Mike, I felt resolute in my new outlook, almost eager to confront the storm again. Almost, but not quite.

When we pulled out again, I screamed out loud to myself, "It's only seventy-five kilometres this time, Heidi! You got this!"

Somehow the rain had gotten even heavier, and the wind felt like an arctic gale dead set on blowing us off the highway. But I couldn't let my mind focus on that. I needed a distraction.

I decided to start talking to Mike about everything and anything. We chatted about friends, movies, and our kids. I knew I had to keep talking. His voice was very comforting inside my helmet.

By the time we arrived at the next rest stop, I was shivering so uncontrollably I could hardly sip my coffee without spilling it.

"Are you okay to keep going?" Mike asked.

"I'm fine," I said. My teeth chattered as I spoke.

Mike grabbed my frozen hand and gave it a reassuring squeeze. "It's only seventy kilometres to the next stop. We're almost home, Heidi."

"How far is it to the house?"

"It's about one hundred and twenty kilometres," he answered.

I sat for a minute and stared into my coffee cup, watching as the steam floated up and disappeared. I took a deep breath, looked up, and said, "Let's not stop. I can do it!"

As I climbed back on the bike, I knew the next hour and a half was going to be torture. I was soaked, freezing, and exhausted from shivering. But I knew it was mind over matter, and I wasn't giving up. The storm would break before I did.

Ten minutes down the highway, Mike asked me how I was doing. I hadn't spoken a word since the last stop, and my jaw was trembling so much I could hardly answer him. "Good" was all I could get out.

As we approached the next rest stop, Mike asked me if I wanted to take one last break. I desperately needed to get warm, but I knew I had to keep going. I answered him with an emphatic *no*.

As we drove past the stop, I felt an amazing euphoria wash over me. I knew the ride was almost over now. My heart started racing. I felt invigorated!

The next forty minutes flew by, and before I knew it, we had pulled into the driveway.

Home at last. It was over. I did it!

So I turn to my sister and say, "No matter what circumstance you're dealing with, whether it's a health issue or any other situation life throws at you, you just have to handle it bit by bit. When you take your problems and break them up into bite-sized little chunks, it's amazing how things that were once so daunting can suddenly seem so manageable.

"Just live one hurdle at a time, one chapter at a time, one day at a time. No matter what journey you're on, set your odometer and only focus on getting to the next rest stop. One day you'll arrive at your destination. Whatever you do, keep riding."

Heidi Allen is the founder of The Positive People Army. It started out as a blog but soon shifted into a movement. Watch out for Heidi's new book, *Stories: Finding Your Wings*.

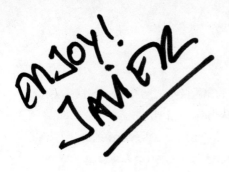
Enjoy! Javier

SODA WATER AND LIME

Javier Vargas

I HIT ROCK BOTTOM—*yet again*. I have a problem, I can't fix myself, and I need help or I will die. The pills my family doctor prescribed for me aren't working, and the desire to trade them in for a few bottles of vodka and some cocaine is back. I haven't had this feeling for a while, and I don't want to relapse. I feel like I am on a plane that is about to crash.

I sign up for an eight-week inpatient treatment-centre program. *Let's do this*, I tell myself as I walk through the front doors. I go to the front desk. "I'm here to check in," I say.

I am more determined this time. I am all too familiar with hospital and rehab stays. But this is different—I am in full-recovery mode. I am learning revolutionary life skills that change the way I experience my feelings and thoughts. I have let my feelings define me all my life; I am *not* depression. I simply suffer from this condition, but it is not who I am.

I sit in my psychiatrist's office. "You do suffer from acute depression and suicidal ideation, but you're not schizophrenic. You are just very, very hard on yourself, and that's where the negative self-talk comes from."

"I'm not schizophrenic?!" I excitedly ask. I can't believe I have been misdiagnosed. This sheds new light into my understanding.

"Well, that's one less thing I have to worry about. Thank you, doctor."

"Yes . . ." he continues, hesitating. "But have you ever been tested for ADHD?"

My excitement is a bit premature, I guess.

I test and add the diagnosis of ADHD to my list. At least I know what my problem is. Once you can name an issue, you can deal with it.

Things are going well, but there is a nagging thought that keeps popping into my mind. I push it aside until a nurse approaches me and says aloud, as if she is reading my internal fears, "We are pairing you up with one of the therapists to start working on your return-to-life-and-work plan after you check out from here."

Suddenly, I feel like I am back on that crashing airplane. "Are you okay?" she asks.

I start walking in circles. I try to process the words. I turn to her. "No, I'm not okay." I am assertive. "How can I be okay? In a few weeks from now I'm going to be in the outside world having to deal with a completely new set of problems."

It won't just be about staying sober . . . I will have to stay sober as I manage trying not to be depressed and suicidal again. I won't have this protective bubble of the clinic and the support I have now. My apprehension lies somewhere between being fearful and terrified.

"This is why we prepare you for it well in advance." She tries to calm my racing mind.

How will I handle life without the support groups? How will I handle work? Will I be able to go out with friends again? If they are all drinking, will I be capable of ordering something else? How will I cope?

The therapist and I start working diligently on a plan that will facilitate my reinsertion back into the "real world." The idea of leaving the safety of the clinic remains daunting during the entire process. Part of me wants to stay in this bubble forever, despite the vile hospital food.

We start our meeting. I begin: "I am not afraid of difficult personal work, and I have had my fair share of trauma. I find it hard to trust people. I lived through a civil war in El Salvador, I've had guns pointed at my head, my first sexual experience was abuse, my family practically disowned me because I'm gay . . . you want me to keep going?" I look at her through tears.

"It wasn't your fault," she says. "None of it was your fault. You are holding onto guilt for things that were done *to* you—things that you had no control over."

We continue to work on the return-to-work plan. I take the extra step of presenting it via conference call to my bosses to make sure that we all understand the importance of it. I am grateful for their support.

Leaving day arrives. I pack, I say my goodbyes, and I walk out the same door I entered eight short weeks ago. I am starting a new life that, in many ways, remains unpredictable.

At home, I temporarily feel a little lost and alone, but I prepare to return to work.

"Welcome back, Javier." One of my colleagues pats my shoulder.

"Javier! You're back." Another hugs me.

So many of my colleagues are genuinely excited and happy to see me.

"Let's celebrate," a co-worker suggests.

"Yeah, let's go to the bar downstairs after work."

It is settled. We are going out after the workday is over. My heart quickens, my blood pressure rises, and my synapses fire. I take a deep breath and continue my day.

After work, we get settled at our favourite bar. Our waiter seems to be the king of efficiency as he takes everyone's order with grace and without writing a single thing down. It's my turn. "Hey, buddy, what can I get you?" he asks.

Mouth opens, thoughts process, default is intercepted: I used to order lots of vodka with very little juice. But I have a plan. I want to be healthy. I want to be happy. I want to live.

"A soda water with lots of lime on the side please," I respond.

I will continue with my plan and with my love for life. And, over time, a soda water with lime will become my default order without giving it even a second thought.

Javier Vargas is an account manager at a software company in Toronto. He immigrated to Canada from El Salvador in 2004. He writes a personal blog on his Facebook page, inspired by his rehab treatment in 2016 and his stay in 2018 at a treatment facility for depression, suicidal ideation, and ADHD. He calls Canada home, and he continues to work on his recovery, living life one day at a time.

PART III

REVOLUTION

rev·o·lu·tion
[rev-uh-loo-shuh n]

a sudden, complete, or marked change in
something

a fundamental change in the way of thinking
about or visualizing something: a change of
paradigm

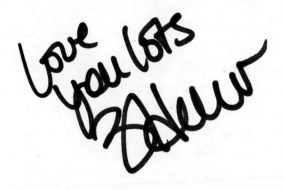

LADYBUG

Natalie Harris

A FELLOW PARAMEDIC AND FRIEND of mine died by suicide in 2014. At his memorial we were told that when he was little, he wanted to be a ladybug when he grew up—and so began my friendship with those little flying beetles. Whenever I see one, I feel like he is there, telling me that he's okay and that I will be okay, too. You see, I am a suicide survivor—I'm not sure how I am here on this planet to type these words. In memory of my friend, I work with politicians to lobby for legislation that will improve the mental health care of first responders, and I was invited to testify on May 16 for the Canadian Standing Committee on Health in Ottawa on Parliament Hill. You would think that, because I have been speaking at conferences, corporate events, and first responder services for approximately two years about my recovery from post-traumatic stress injury, I would be confident in my ability to provide a detailed and an impactful account of my struggle, but on this particular day, I was riddled with anxiety about this invitation.

I wake up not feeling rested. It's such an important day . . . and I feel like crap. Exhausted from the four-hour drive the day before and from socializing beyond my anxiety limit the night before,

I am walking in a fog of hangover proportions—without the alcohol. Sigh. I make my way to Parliament Hill with my friend and moral support, Heather, with coffee-free blood pumping through my veins. I'm irritable. Every sound I hear makes my eardrums bounce with pain. *I will be okay*, I keep telling myself. But truly I am not sure how I'm going to hold it all together when I am already this stressed before noon.

"You got this!" says Heather with the kindness she always has in her voice.

"I need a sign. Something to show me that things will be okay." I am big on trusting that the universe has me and that when I need a sign, it gets sent directly to me.

"I bet we meet the prime minister today. You want to know why?" continues Heather. "Because I have no makeup on. I bet you we meet him when I look like *this*." We both chuckle at the unlikely possibility.

We park in what feels like provinces away from Parliament Hill, and I resign myself to the fact that I will most likely get a second wind. The cold breeze we walk through will perk me up.

"I really need coffee," I say again to poor Heather.

The testimony gets under way. I have a bag beside me with my paramedic dress uniform in it. I may be using it today. Not to wear—for something much more important. I begin my testimony.

Good morning honourable members of Parliament and their staff, members of the Standing Committee on Health, analysts, proceedings and verification officer, and honourable chairperson. My name is Natalie Harris, and it is my pleasure to have this opportunity to share with you how important Bill C-211, introduced by MP Todd Doherty, is to me and to so many first responders, veterans, military personnel, and corrections officers across Canada. Establishing a national framework to address the challenges of recognizing the symptoms and providing timely diagnosis and treatment of post-traumatic stress is essential to saving the lives of those who passionately care for and protect the citizens of this great country every day.

You may be thinking to yourselves, "What in the world could this seemingly normal girl possibly teach me today?" Well, I may not be representing an organization, but that's okay, because what I do represent is very important. I stand here before you, representing what could be your sister, mother, daughter, wife, friend, or partner who may be silently battling a world of darkness all on their own because they are too afraid to ask for help for fear of no longer being able to do the job they so dearly love—for fear of being ridiculed, labelled, and not being heard.

In October 2014, post-traumatic stress had caused me to live in a world filled with fear and sadness that constantly undervalued my fundamental necessity to breathe. It caused me to live in a world filled with darkness, distorted thinking, and illogical reasoning. It caused me to live in a world that harboured powerful voices who told me that I should hurt myself because I was worthless and that everyone would be better off without me. In October 2014, PTSD caused me to know for certain that I was going to take my own life.

On that dreaded day, after swallowing half a bottle of muscle relaxants, I wrote a letter to whomever would find me: *I'm so sorry. You will be okay. I love you.* I then swallowed the rest of the bottle. I started to feel tired; I knew the medicine was working. I lay in bed staring at the ceiling, more numb than I'd ever been in my life . . . while I was waiting to die. I remember feeling sick and somehow in my haze made it to the bathroom . . . and that's all I remember that day. For all I knew, I would never wake up again. For all I knew, I was dead. What I didn't know was that my colleagues had found me and brought me to the hospital, where I remained unconscious for twelve hours. The doctors and nurses pumped litres of fluid into me with the hope of saving my liver. As the hours went by, my abdomen grew full of fluid, and I turned jaundiced as evidence that my liver couldn't keep up. My family and friends were seriously discussing funeral plans for me. But somehow—*somehow!*—I survived. It wasn't time for me to leave this planet quite yet. I still had some pretty important work to do, which has brought me here today.

Over the years while being a full-time paramedic, I literally became very comfortable with uncomfortable. I became acclimatized to live a life that included horrific memories, relentless nightmares, and engrained images of sadness and pain. That may sound barbaric to anyone not in the emergency services field, but it's literally part of our almost daily lives. Devil's advocates out there may be saying to themselves that we signed up for it, but we didn't. We signed up for an amazing career that allows us to help people on such an extraordinary level; no one signed up for mental turmoil. We signed up for the chance to save people's lives; no one signed up for memories of patients screaming in pain. We signed up for achieving educational goals; no one signed up for drowning our sorrows in vices. We thought we would be strong enough to avoid being uncomfortable; but no one is. Strength isn't measured by the number of deaths we pronounce. It's measured by the number of deaths we recognized we need to talk about in order to sleep at night. First responders are amazing people. But signing up to be one didn't mean we signed away our hearts.

It's not normal to have a person ask you to just take their leg and arm off because they were experiencing so much pain from being trapped in a car while having multiple open fractures all over their body. It's not normal to learn that the patient who hanged himself the night before had a second noose waiting for his wife had his son not called 9-1-1 in time. It's not normal to witness a young woman, seven months pregnant, rub her belly with the only limb that could move as she had a stroke that would leave her disabled. It's not normal to see the cellphone on the road beside the obviously dead driver crushed between the pavement and the car who was texting and driving—and it's not normal to know he made the three sisters in the other car now two. It's not normal to experience and see the look of true evil when you learn how two innocent women were murdered. It's not normal to be handed a baby that's blue. It's not normal to watch a child have a seizure for thirty minutes because the drugs just wouldn't work. It's not normal to watch people die right before your very eyes more times than you could count. What we do isn't normal, so why would we think it's okay to act comfortable with that? Why would it be any surprise to hear that first responders are dying every month because they can't take their often-hidden memories any longer? I'm uncomfortable with how comfortable we've become.

Honourable members of the committee, we can't wait any longer to acknowledge and act upon the cries of heroes and their families, which are happening right now coast to coast. They need Canada to step up to the plate and value their sacrifices in the form of education and support. So much more needs to be done to prevent the deaths of our community heroes, and Bill C-211 is where this can start! It's on the table. We can't push it aside. If we do, time wasted will equal lives lost.

I would like to end my testimony by sharing a poem that I wrote in memory of my colleague, who died by suicide in September 2014. I miss him and will never forget him.

I read the poem, then I reach for my dress uniform, hands shaking but proud. I continue my testimony.

I never had the opportunity to choose to hang up my uniform; sadly PTSD made that decision for me. I plead of you today to move this bill forward and put Canada on the map with respect to having the best national framework for our heroes so that every uniform can be hung up when the time is right—with the hero's choice.

The testimony ends with questions. I leave feeling that I made a difference, but I still didn't get the sign I was hoping for.

We are invited to observe question period by our local representative, John Brassard. Then, the head of the Standing Health Committee, Bill Casey, introduces us to the prime minister. Heather gets *her* sign today. But where is mine?

We head back to the home where we are staying and take time to admire the numerous beautiful pieces of artwork our host has created. When I enter her painting room, I am in awe of the colours and textures in her work. But there's something else that catches my eye—a painting of two ladybugs, nose to nose, in a heart. Tears fill my eyes. I try to wipe them away quickly, but my host recognizes that there is something wrong with me and asks if I'm okay. I explain to her the importance of the ladybug, and she smiles ear to ear.

"Natalie, this isn't the only ladybug in this house. There is one hiding in every piece of artwork I have made."

My sign! I had been surrounded by ladybugs this whole time. I immediately feel at peace. My friend Bob has been with me all day, and I didn't even know it.

"I was meant to stay here," I say to my host, and wipe the endless tears from my eyes. *Things are going to be okay*, I think. *Yes, things are definitely going to be okay.*

Over a year later, I am in Ottawa again. This time with my daughter, Caroline. Bill C-211 has reached royal assent, and I am attending the reception the day before. After the assent the next day, we travel back home. As I am scrolling through Facebook, a post catches my eye. It is a picture of a hand-written note:

Todd,

I would like to congratulate you on the passage of Bill C-211.

On May 16, 2007, the Standing Committee on Health received this uniform, worn by Ms. Natalie Harris. As Chair of this committee, it gives me great pleasure to present you with Ms. Harris' uniform as a token and a symbol of your hard work for first responders.

Sincerely,

Bill Casey

My heart skips a beat; I scroll to the next picture: *my uniform*, adjusting to its new permanent home on Parliament Hill. *Things are okay*, I think. *They really are.*

Natalie Harris is the mother of furbabies and real people. She writes for *Huffington Post Canada*. You can follow her on Twitter @paramedicnat1.

ZACH MAKES TRACKS

Zach Hofer

IT IS DAY 12 OF my trip between Barrie and Ottawa, Ontario. I am walking, running, and biking my way across the province to raise money and awareness for youth mental health. Tired, I push the pedal down on my bike with all my might as I inch up the hill. "Keep closer to the line," Derek, my stepdad, yells at me as he pedals beside me.

"Why do I have to stay so close to the line?" I complain. Everything hurts, and Derek is being so annoying.

"You need to ride safely. There is traffic."

Isn't that what the police escort is for? I think.

I ignore his comment. "Why are there so many hills?" I mutter.

"Pardon?" Derek chimes in. He is getting on my nerves.

"Nothing. Are there no signs to say how far the next town is? Why don't they have any signs? This is stupid. I am going to write a letter to every mayor and complain. They need more signs."

"It's not stupid, Zach. Just try to focus on why you are doing this."

Last straw.

"And, Derek, speaking of stupid things. Why do you always get mad at me for putting my elbows on the table? Seriously, why is that such a big deal? I don't get it." I am now officially mad.

Right now, I want to be anywhere but here. Just last week, country-singer Trevor Panczak stopped me on my journey and asked if he could get a selfie with *me*. Shouldn't it be the other way around? I am only thirteen. I'm exhausted from all of the attention, I'm tired of the pressure, and I sure hate these hills. Why is it so hilly here? I wish that when I first had this idea, I had worn a mask. That way, I could be invisible.

In the beginning, it seemed like a good idea. I had always idolized Terry Fox and really wanted to do something to help youth and mental health. I have a family member who has mental illness and some friends at school, too. I had no idea that the plan would grow and gain so much attention. I never expected that I would be doing TV appearances all the time, or having reporters interview me, or that I would get to meet so many famous people. And I never imagined that this campaign would generate over one hundred thousand dollars. But in this moment, I don't care. I want to stop. I want to go home and sit in my room and play video games for an entire week straight.

"Boy, you are extra negative today," Derek offers. "I know it's hard. I really hurt, too. Remember, I'm doing this as well."

I don't think he understands the pressure I am under. "Yeah, but you can quit anytime you want to. It isn't *Derek* Makes Tracks, is it?"

We stop arguing because we are no longer speaking to each other. I am mad and so is he.

I can't do it anymore. I stop pedalling and go over to the side of the road.

Derek stops as well and comes over to me. "I promised your mom and your dad that I would be beside you every single kilometre, taking care of you and making sure you were safe so that you could finish strong in Ottawa."

My mom joins us. Before I started the journey, I was asked to do a lot of public speaking. I would get anxious and nervous, and at the time my mom didn't want to share that on social media in hopes of giving a positive appearance for the campaign. But I didn't want to pretend to be something I'm not—she really didn't either. We both learned that being honest was better, anyway. Lots of people could relate to my anxiety and would reach out to us if we were having challenges. So we had an agreement to share not only the good times but our struggles as well.

"I posted a picture on Facebook, Twitter, and Instagram, Zach." She shows me the shot. It is me, angry, at the side of the road with my head down. "I let your followers know that you are struggling."

I don't say anything. I am not ready to talk to anyone yet.

My mom continues. "Here are some of the things people are saying . . ."

My mom starts to read the comments aloud. Thank you, Zach, for digging deep and pushing through for all the kids who can't, like my own son, who has suffered with mental illness for years and has been hospitalized once . . .

And then another. Don't quit, Zach. You can do it—you're stronger than your frustration. Keep it up!

My mom keeps reading comment after comment. I hear the words and feel the encouragement. I am quiet. I am tired. I am just a kid. But I can also prove that you don't have to be the loudest person in the room to make the biggest impact. Slowly, my legs feel a bit better, and I realize that I should continue, that I *want* to continue. I can do this—not just for the people cheering me on or for the people donating money for mental health, but for *me*.

I get back on the bike and push forward, Derek by my side. We aren't talking much, but we aren't arguing either.

At the end of the day, we end up back in our RV at the resort. I'm in my bunk, watching my TV. I am tired, but I am also happy . . . and proud. I am proud I pushed through. I know we probably didn't go as far as we usually did, but at least I finished the day. Just like people suffering with mental illness, sometimes you can't avoid your problems, you just have to face them head on. I realize I can't wear a mask while doing this trip, just like those trying to tell their honest mental health stories also have to be mask-free.

Derek is calculating the distance we covered today.

"Guess what?" he asks me. I don't have a chance to answer before he continues. "We travelled the farthest distance in a single day to date!"

So true, I think, *not just in kilometres, but in understanding*. My favourite saying is REACH FOR THE MOON. EVEN IF YOU MISS, YOU'LL LAND AMONG THE STARS. I feel like I touched a star today.

Today is a turning point. Because I pushed through the hills and fatigue, I am stronger and more confident. I don't know it yet, but I won't have any more days nearly as bad as this one. I will continue on to finish my trip, on time, ending up in Canada's capital city. I will meet the prime minister and many others who followed my journey, and I will realize that the struggles are just as important as the good times.

Zach Hofer is a fourteen-year-old teenager from Barrie, Ontario. In 2017, Zach wanted to help kids who were struggling with mental health and rallied his community to raise over $110,000 for the Youth Mental Health unit at his local hospital by walking, running, and biking from Barrie to Ottawa. He loves basketball, bouldering, and hanging with friends. Although he tells a great joke, he doesn't like being in the spotlight. But he did it anyway to make a difference for the kids in the region.

ONE HOOF AT A TIME

Maud Revel

TECHNICALLY, I TEACH FRENCH TO the Canadian Armed Forces. However, sometimes a job is more than its title.

The military consists of more than infantry, officers, and non-officers: There are also dentists, nurses, medics, firefighters, police officers, drivers, mechanics, cooks, and many other professions. I enjoy being able to work with many diverse adult learners from all walks of life.

I invite a guest speaker to address the class one day. "Good afternoon, class. I am excited to announce that you won't have to listen to me today. Instead, I have brought a guest to share his experiences overseas—in French, of course."

A few weak laughs. The class knows the presentation couldn't possibly be in English!

As my guest begins to share his interesting presentation, most students sit, attentive and polite. Except one. Instead of paying attention, he stares out the window, playing with a pen on his desk. He doesn't even look at the speaker once during the entire presentation. I feel slightly uncomfortable, a little embarrassed even, that my guest has to witness this. *This is disrespectful*, I think to myself.

But I still have a lot to learn, a lot to understand, and more importantly, a lot to do about what I witness.

Part of the French training I offer my classes includes regular one-on-one meetings with each student. I meet with the "disrespectful" student. As he is an adult learner, I am careful to treat him with dignity and courtesy, so I do not bring up his questionable behaviour right away. As it turns out, I don't need to. We talk about other subjects and he breaks down.

"The nightmares . . ." he starts, the weight of his memories bringing him to tears. His personal battles spill out, unfiltered and uncontrolled.

"I can't do this alone." He continues, "I need help to deal with my demons."

I am dumbfounded. I don't know how to react.

This big, burly soldier is still processing trauma from a previous mission. I realize in this moment that his behaviour is not a lack of deference for my course but simply a coping mechanism to deal with his post-traumatic stress.

I reach out to learn more about post-traumatic stress. I am able to notice the signs in my students faster with time and experience. Although I am not trained in the mental health field, my common sense and instincts serve me well, and I am able to work with students to better accommodate their needs so that they can learn the language more efficiently.

I am happy with my new understanding, but I want to do more to help. However, I simply don't know what.

Years go by, and I am invited to a formal mess hall dinner. During the meal, I excuse myself.

"Where is my seat?" I ask when I return.

"I don't know," my colleague answers.

"No idea," another chimes in. However, I notice the corners of her mouth turn upward.

I try to continue the night—evening gown and high heels be damned—pretending to sit at the table without a chair. I will not become the focus of the evening.

Luckily, someone has pity on me and returns my chair after a few minutes. "Don't you know that in old military tradition, if you leave the table before dinner is finished, you lose your chair?"

"I do now . . ."

It seems learning experiences are my lot in life.

I am excited to listen to the speaker, Major (retired) Dee Brasseur. She is one of the first three female pilots in the Canadian Armed Forces, one of the first two female CF-18 fighter pilots, and Canada's first female aircraft accident investigator.

During her inspirational speech, she promotes the use of service dogs for military members affected by PTSD. I am intrigued. It is a lightbulb moment.

I grew up in the land of cheese, apples, and horses: Normandy, France. When I was sixteen, my parents shipped me off to England for two weeks. I almost didn't go because my horse had injured himself a few days before I was scheduled to catch the ferry. I desperately wanted to stay back to take care of him. However, my parents didn't see it that way. To them, learning to speak English was a more important task. Someone else could look after my horse in my absence.

Reluctantly, I went off to England, and I had a blast. The family I stayed with had two horses. They took me to Oxford. We toured around. They trusted me with the tea-making ritual—a very serious mix of fifty percent Lapsang Souchong and fifty percent Ceylon. We even went to Alton Towers amusement park. (Truth or dare happened a few times. I dared. And the truth is, I will never go back on a ride—ever.)

Two years later, I ended up in Australia to meet an estranged branch of my family. Then I found a job in Ireland, working at a busy riding school. Initially, I was hired to muck stalls, but one day my boss asked me to ride a horse named Prince once before handing him over to clients. I tacked him up and walked to the arena. I got on, and he turned into a bucking bronco. As I experienced this impromptu rodeo session, the boss ran into the yard and yelled at me. I couldn't catch what she said.

"Can you repeat that?" I asked.

"Get off that horse right now!" she screamed.

But I was the one in control here, not the horse, and I did not give up easily. I intended to win the first round of this rodeo. Finally, the horse stopped bucking, and he turned into the best riding school horse: quiet, placid, smooth under saddle. I took him down to the beach and back without issue. Then I hopped off. I am sure that I won a few points with my boss because I started to ride more horses; I was even asked to lead a couple of beach rides. And two weeks later when the lead trail guide quit his job, I was promoted to trail guide. Best summer ever—five-mile beach as a playground, riding three to six hours per day for six days a week.

My love of horses and my travel bug continued to flourish. Eventually, I ended up in Canada, enrolling in a master's program. My wandering days came to an end, however, when I met my special someone.

Now I teach French at a military base.

As I sit in this room, listening to Dee Brasseur's presentation, the seeds of an idea are being planted.

At the end of the evening, I make my way to our guest of honour.

"Thank you for your presentation," I venture. "I enjoyed it. You are very inspirational. I have a question."

"Thank you. I would love to hear your question."

"Have you ever heard of people using horses instead of dogs to help ground people with PTSD?"

"Yes, yes, I have heard of people doing this. Although I have not been engaged with or participated in anything like that, it is certainly out there."

"Just listening to you tonight, I thought it would be a great service to offer. I absolutely love horses, and working with the military for the past few years has led me to want to help those suffering with PTSD. I would be very interested in trying to create and run a program using horses."

Then the words that cement the idea into concrete action: "If you think you can do it, just go for it," she answers.

Hearing that encouragement and reinforcement of my initial idea from such an accomplished individual is nothing short of inspiring.

"Welcome to the inaugural session at New Horserizons." I address the very first group of participants in my equine assisted learning class a few months later—research, certification, curriculum development, location, and sponsorship all water under the bridge. I look at the participants, mostly former French students willing to do a trial run for my brand new company, and I am filled with such joy. Their feedback is fantastic.

Over the next two years, many more people attend my program. I meet first responders, police officers, firefighters, nurses, dispatchers—they all fight the same battle.

I see people revolutionized by the power of connection and the potential of teamwork. I see people go from shy to confident, fearful to trusting, reticent to jumping out of their comfort zone. This is where I thrive. People thank me for running this program for them, but I thank them for trusting me. I feel a little selfish because I feed off their progress and am honoured to be part of their journey. I know the road is long and sometimes dark, and I am grateful that my horses bring a little bit of light to their day.

Maud Revel was born and raised in France. She has studied sciences, history, and languages in France, Ireland, Germany, and Canada. She holds a master of arts with a focus on Irish history and translation of popular literature. She is a French language teacher at CFB Borden and a certified equine assisted learning facilitator. She owns NEW HOrseRIZONS and runs EAL programs out of Brentwood, Ontario. When not at work or at the barn, she enjoys reading and hiking (in good weather). Connect via email at newhorserizons@gmail.com or Facebook @newhorserizons.

Enjoy!

Christine

WHADDAYA SAY WE

Christine Newman

I AM LYING AWAKE IN bed when my alarm rings. *Good grief. People get up at this hour every day?* I think as I force myself out of bed at four a.m. to get ready for an interview with Matt Galloway, the host of CBC Radio's *Metro Morning*.

I look at myself in the mirror while I brush my teeth; my mind runs through the day's events. *Going to be a busy day*, I surmise as I climb into the shower. I find I do a lot of thinking in the shower. It is an automatic series of functions, so I can let my mind run free to ponder other topics. This morning, I look back at over thirty years of LGBTQ activism and advocacy work, wondering how someone who spends most of her time working behind the scenes is now a go-to person for discussing issues affecting trans folks or the larger LGBTQ community. Interesting how these things work out.

As I tiptoe from the bathroom to my bedroom, I remind myself, *Remember to not drop any f-bombs on the air, be short, to the point, concise but not terse, just have a conversation with Matt.* The main thing we will be discussing is the introduction of Bill C-16 in Parliament today—whether the Trans Rights Bill, something that has failed numerous times in the past, will be the one that makes it. But holy cow, this will be simulcast locally on

CBC television at the time we're going to be having this chat on air . . . and oh my God, the audience is around one million people. *Skip that, just talk with the people who are in the studio, I remind myself.* One more glance at the clock. *Okay lady, get it in gear, time's a-wasting! Don't forget to bring your bookbag. You'll have three more events this morning before you get a chance to pop home to change.* "Okay, got that," I answer myself aloud.

As I lock the door to my apartment at five a.m., I remember my mom. We always did this thing. I would say to her, "One day, Mom, I'll make you proud, promise." Me, on the radio, live on air on Toronto's number one morning show—yes she would be proud of me today. I'm making good time on the walk to the CBC building, keeping in mind that they told me to be at the security desk in the lobby for five-thirty a.m. so that I have time to relax in the green room before going on air just after six o'clock. I check my watch anyway. Force of habit. *Plenty of time still*, and my mind begins to replay memories of my mom, good memories, as I walk along the street.

Given the opportunity, I will regale folks for hours with the hilarious stories of our adventures and antics over the years— particularly when it came to Mom's '69 Volkswagen Beetle named Betsy. Although, when acting up and being temperamental, Betsy was known by much more colourful names, as you can imagine. We delivered phone books; they came in packs of ten, weighing fifty pounds. One hundred and fifty books could be crammed into every available space in that car. It was something to do while off work recovering from surgery. In the winter, everybody in the car would hold an ice scraper to keep all the windows clear because the standard heater had, as was typical at the time, rusted out and fallen off after two years, and the gas heater would drain the tank in thirty minutes flat. During the days of full-service gas stations, the VW Bug was not a common car. Mom would pull in, tell the attendant to fill it up, and ask if they could please check the oil, too. Inevitably, before she could explain where the engine was (in the rear on the original models), they would have their hand on the front trunk-lid, telling her to unlock the hood. Mom reached into the glove compartment and pulled the lever down to unlock it, and they would stand there with the hood up—some for a few seconds, some for a few minutes—before looking around the hood and saying, "Where's the engine, lady?" Mom sat there trying desperately not to laugh at them while she explained that she was trying to tell them that the engine was in the rear.

I could entertain you with tales of the hilarity we got up to, because we did have adventures, the two of us. Adventures with Mom always began with her saying "Whaddaya say we . . ." and ended with "just for the hell of it?" And one side-eye glance with a twinkle in her eye meant that she was about to say something classic and hilarious, funny to the point you would laugh until tears were streaming down your face and you were gasping for air in between the laughs, particularly if she had thought of something risqué—that would be my cue to look at her in feigned shock while exclaiming, "Mother!" She would then put on her most innocent look and say, "What?" right before we both cracked up and roared with laughter. I'm telling you, life was never dull wherever the two of us were.

I think of the year Mom took a part-time job at Eaton's Yorkdale to make some extra cash for Christmas shopping, working in the ladies department. This was at the time when pantsuits had become all the rage. Mom arrived home late and could not wait to share the tales from the sales floor that night. Think of the British comedy *Are You Being Served?* to get an idea of life as a sales clerk in a large department store. She said this woman came in minutes before closing time, and all the full-timers ran and hid behind racks of clothing and left the part-timer to serve her. Picture the snobbiest woman you can, mink coat to the floor, dripping in jewels, and the attitude to go with it, too. Madam snapped her fingers at Mom (*huge* mistake!—that's like waving a red cape in front of a pissed-off bull) and barked at her, "Bring me pantsuits. I must have pantsuits!" Mom looked through the sizes on the racks and took selections into a change room for Madam. She said that Madam emerged, red-faced and raging, calling her incompetent and stupid. Mom said Madam finally shut up for a second, and Mom quietly said to her while looking over her glasses, "The reason that the pants are so baggy in the front like that is that you have put them on backwards. Perhaps Madam is not aware that the labels inside are meant to go over your ass."

Madam fled to the change room, and when she re-emerged, flung the pantsuits, hangers and all, on the sales desk, threw her Eaton's card at Mom, and said, "I'll take them all." Mom tried desperately not to laugh while ringing this up, because she could hear the giggles sneaking out from behind the racks where the full-timers were hiding. She handed Madam the bag with the pantsuits, her card, and the bill. The woman turned without saying a word and stomped out of the store to gales of laughter that erupted as soon as she snatched the bag from Mom's hand. Mom had one parting shot after Madam was well out of earshot: "I wonder who pissed in her cornflakes this morning?" Everybody howled with laughter again.

As I'm crossing University Avenue, I think about how fast the tables would turn. Mom's diagnosis of terminal brain cancer (glioblastoma multiforme) at the start of 2010 would mean that we would switch roles without even thinking about it. As her cancer progressed—the way it erased her mind backwards—it ended up fitting that, as she became my child, I became her mother, her nurse, her doctor, and the person who got up in the middle of the night when she was hungry. I would make something for her to snack on (eating was always a win at that time!). I took on that role willingly, without any hesitation; it was the natural thing to do. People we knew said to me, "Why do you go to the hospital every single day?" And as I would explain many times over those seven months that she had left, anytime I was sick, if I woke up feverish or worse in the middle of the night, she was always sitting by the bed reading while keeping watch. If I was in the hospital recovering from surgery, she was the last face I saw before going into surgery and the first person I saw every time I opened my eyes when I was back in my room. She was the one I could always count on to drop everything and come running when needed. It was my turn to pay it back, and that's why I was at her side every minute that she was awake or aware. She had beaten ovarian and uterine cancer, had defeated breast cancer, but this time there was no win—we already knew how the fight would end, and I would be there holding her hand when she drew her final breath.

I miss her terribly. She wasn't able to be there when I became homeless or when I was beaten within an inch of my life, or survived two suicide attempts, or when my post-traumatic stress disorder, anxiety, and depression became almost too much to bear. I wish she was still with me physically. Yet in many ways, she has made her presence known to me many times since her death.

I arrive at the CBC building and find the entrance door mentioned in the email.

I walk up to the security desk, and this gent looks like he's already at his limits in the final hours of the overnight shift. In my mind, I say to Mom, *Just watch me*, with a saucy wink.

"Morning, Sunshine! Christine Newman. I'm here for *Metro Morning*. Where do you need me to sign? You can tell me where to go, just be gentle, okay?" Success! Not only does he smile, he lets out a little chuckle . . . gotcha! He asks, "Have you seen the other guest who will be on air with you this morning?"

"Nope. Just little old me," I answer.

I sign in, and he hands me a security pass. "Use that pass to go through that gate to your left, and there are elevators around that corner once you go through. Take an elevator up to four. One of the producers will meet you there." I flash him a smile and a wink, and I'm off on an adventure! I've never done this before, and I look like a tourist seeing things for the first time.

I remember this lovely young woman, Taylor, the producer who had booked me for this and had conducted the pre-interview over the phone. Taylor met me at the elevator and ushered me into the green room, showed me the coffee (YAY!), and would be back to go over the questions Matt would ask that morning. I'm sitting there taking in all the sights and thinking, *Good. I'm not late. Glad I left early and got here when they asked me to.*

The other guest I am going to be on air with blows through the door breathlessly with just minutes to spare. We are supposed to be ready to go on air live just after six a.m. She takes one look at me and exclaims in abject horror, "Oh my God, you have no makeup on! Do you not realize this is simulcast live on TV in HD?!"

I look over my glasses at her and reply, "Honey, it is barely six a.m. I have been up since four, and at this time of the morning, you're bloody lucky I remembered to put clothes on. I'm in my fifties for chrissake. If they wanted cute, they can always hire a model! But they called for an opinionated old broad to talk on the radio, and here I am!"

Laughter erupts from the producers in the doorway of the green room. In that moment of spontaneous wit, I hear my mother's voice. As has happened so many times since losing her, I have opened my mouth and classic Joyce has come rolling out. I realize that I can't miss my mom, not really, because her influence and sense of humour will not—*cannot*—ever leave me.

I drain the last bit of coffee from the cup, and after a quick reminder of what the questions should be, we head into the studio. I'm doing my tourist thing again, looking at all the television cameras and screens, all the equipment, looking behind me into the control room at the people and all the flashing lights. *Holy cow*, I think. *Looks like we're doing this!*

Matt introduces himself, shakes our hands, and takes a photo that he tweets out announcing we are up next, and we settle in and watch Toronto's most popular morning show happen all around us. I'll just bet Mom is sitting somewhere watching this, grinning from ear to ear. And as Matt starts the introduction to our segment, I settle in for a conversation, tuning out everything happening around me.

I had told a few friends that I would be on air that morning. It was one more conversation before C-16 would be introduced in Parliament that day. I had been given a preview of the wording, so I knew what things I wanted to touch on that day, but most of all, I wanted to discuss hope—look at the progress made over the decades, the changes I had seen in thirty-four years of advocacy work at that time. Then I mentioned the work I do with the Toronto Police. Matt said, "I want to discuss that further, right after this." It's just the work I've been doing for years. I often forget that it is a big thing for a transgender woman to work with police in causing change to happen. Matt tells the control room he is going to continue with this, and we're back live on air. As we wrap up the conversation, I mention once again the hope that I have today. As they go to break and we are getting up from our chairs to leave, Matt shakes my hand and says, "Anytime you would like to come back and talk more about your work, please let us know."

I'm not really paying much attention to the other guest talking to the producer as we walk back to the elevators. Just like Mom, I have two great desires in life at this moment: the biggest coffee I can find and a cigarette . . . or three. As we reach the lobby door, I say my farewells. "Thanks for the offer of a ride, but I have to go in multiple directions quickly."

I head off in search of coffee and cigarettes, which are right by the subway station where I need to board the west-bound train in order to head toward two high school assemblies. I'm walking along as the streets are coming to life with the first hint of rush hour. It's just hit six-thirty a.m., and I take my phone out of my purse to see what was going on while I was in the CBC building.

Yikes! My notifications have gone wild, and I'm scrolling through screen after screen of tweets, emails, text messages, and more. The few friends I had told that I would be on air spread the news, and a few of the officers I work with at Toronto Police had been live-tweeting my interview. I feel a hand on my shoulder and I spin around, but there is not a soul there. Ahh . . .

The kid did good, eh, Mom? I swear I hear, "Nice work, Kit. I'm proud of you," come back.

I would do more on-air interviews at other radio stations throughout the afternoon, but I am still beaming about *Metro Morning.* I am asked to return that afternoon to tape an interview for the *News at Six*, continuing the conversation begun on *Metro Morning.* In the months that follow, I would be interviewed on CBC's *The National* and tape a segment that would be used in the Canada Day broadcast.

For most of my life, I had a deadly fear of being in front of a camera or behind a microphone—do not, will not, could not, ain't gonna happen. If you want to see my anxiety redline, put me in that situation, and I will go rigid and mute, with a thousand-mile stare. I can stand and deliver a three-hour lecture in a classroom, but throw in a microphone or camera, and I shut down completely.

What changed? A conversation I had with a treasured friend who had given my name and contact information to the producers at *Metro Morning.* She said, "Christine, you know I love you, and I would not ask you to do anything that makes you uncomfortable. I am asking you to trust me, that you can do this, that your voice needs to be heard, that we all need to be visible, that we have a good chance this time of being allowed to exist. I will be at a television station having the same conversation you will be having on the radio. Whaddaya say we do this together, just for the hell of it?"

Did you see it? Yes. "Whaddaya say we . . . just for the hell of it?" That was when I overcame that lifelong fear. I found the day that I could keep my promise. I made you proud, Mom.

Christine Newman is a writer and visiting guest-lecturer based in Toronto. She has been an LGBTQ activist and advocate for thirty-six years and an advocate in the field of mental health/illness/injury for over twenty years, focused on PTSD and first responder mental health and peer support. She writes about her own life, sharing the teachable moments to help others understand.

DELETED

Jeff Emmerson

I LOOK AT THE SCREEN. It reads: Are you sure you want to delete your WordPress account? Like a flash of lightning, I press YES. And just like that, my entire blog about my journey with ADHD is gone. My anxiety wins again, causing me to do something in the heat of the moment, and I regret it already. I am breathing fast and my chest feels like someone is gripping it and twisting it in their hands. My palms are wet and my fingers go numb because I am breathing too quickly. My world is spiralling out of control as anxiety reaches its peak. I begin to cry uncontrollably and wish I were anywhere but inside my own body. It really doesn't matter how many times I have gone through this—it always feels like I am going to die . . . and I'm okay with that. In the throes of anxiety, any escape is welcomed.

Previously, I had lost my brother to suicide, and my world crumbled to pieces. None of us saw it coming. We thought he was okay enough to battle the pain this world can bring, but little did we know that the enemy inside of him—his mind filled with mental illness, frustration, and self-doubt—was much more powerful than we had anticipated. The thought of never seeing him again still makes me physically ill to this day. I miss him so much, but I'm not mad at him. He did not give up; mental illness simply won. His battle shield was broken from fighting the demons for so long, and one final fight was lost because he was unarmed and mangled, not necessarily ready to die, but defeated nonetheless.

I remember the day I wanted to die, too—when my demons were winning. I had no job and my wife was cleaning toilets to help us pay the bills. She is always there for me; this day was no different.

"I can't take it any longer. I feel like I am useless and am letting you down," I said as I cried into my hands.

"Honey, I love you. We will get through this together. I know that you will find your calling. We just need some more time."

"More time is so painful, though," I wailed. "My mind is in constant chaos, and I feel so alone."

"But you're not alone. You have me," my wife said as she reached to hold my hands.

I love her so much and believed her somehow. The demons told me not to, but I did.

Time passes and perspectives change. I sit at my desk, filling in the blanks from when I deleted my work. Today I am writing about friendships and mental health challenges:

> Friendships can be instrumental to a healthy sense of well-being. Feeling connected to others is a wonderful feeling that can play a huge role on our sense of happiness and joy in life. Knowing we've got support from people who care (even if it's only one friend) is like a security blanket we can rely on. However, friends can also be unhealthy for us if the relationship is one based on co-dependency or if one

friend is in a negative spiral of something like addiction or other destructive behaviours, so we need to be aware of our friendships and how healthy they are.

I want to add to this that being your own best friend is something we often aren't taught—the reality that caring for yourself is every bit as important as caring for others is. After all, we can only help others and society to the degree that we take care of ourselves. Burnout happens when you take care of others at the price of your own wellness. People in the care-giving and social work industries know all about this.

No matter what you might have learned, remember this: Taking care of yourself is just as important as helping anyone else.

I am the co-author of *Beyond ADHD*, a mental health start-up founder, and a global mental health advocate, as well as the co-founder of my wife's digital marketing agency. I have found my calling just as my wife had promised. I can never thank her enough for believing in me—for being my rock and for waiting patiently as I navigated my mental health challenges. I may have deleted so much of my previous work while I was being ravaged by anxiety and despair. But that's okay. Today is a new day to share . . . and here I am sharing with you that recovery is possible. Anxiety and ADHD symptoms don't have to rule your life. Pause and think before you press delete—you are worth it. As irony would have it, I now realize that the darkest moments have taught me the most appreciation for life and for the simple things (the most important ones, it turns out).

Born and raised in Ontario, Jeff Emmerson began speaking publicly to raise awareness about mental health and ADHD in 2013, following a suicide attempt and resulting ADHD diagnosis. (Two years earlier, his brother Ryan died by suicide.) In 2013, after committing himself to the locked psych ward of his local hospital for two weeks after again researching ways to end his life, Jeff took to social media channels and began blogging to reach an even larger audience—at which time he began reworking an old manuscript he had written about his life.

He is a passionate advocate for mental health, seeking ways to come up with solutions that return society to a holistic place of compassion, humanity, community, and empathy. For more information, please visit jeffemmerson.com.

POSTPARTUM REPRESSION

Patricia Tomasi

I'M AWAKE. IT'S DARK. That means I shouldn't be awake.

I check my phone. It's midnight. Damn. Why am I awake again?

This better not be. It can't be. I won't let it be.

I look over and check on Celeste. She's still sleeping. Good. I can't deal with an awake three-month-old right now. Not in this state. As long as I don't make too much noise and keep my boob nearby, she should stay asleep.

We co-sleep so I can sleep, because without sleep, I'm a mess. We're a mess. Having her in my bed next to me is easy. Easier. When she stirs, I lean over and guide her quivering lips to my nipple. She suckles herself back to sleep. No crying, no fussing, no rocking, just sleep—sublime, cavernous, essential sleep.

This isn't cute, interesting, or blissful. This is motherhood. This is war. This is exhausting, mundane, and obstreperous. This is a battle of the mind, a battle for *my* mind, and the only way I know how to survive life with a baby.

The house is quiet—well, *almost* quiet. Down the hallway, my husband snores next to my six-year-old in her purple bed, in her purple room, the two of them snuggled under her purple comforter, surrounded by purple walls and dozens of Monster High dolls. I co-slept with Eva until I had Celeste. Now John has taken over. He doesn't mind. His mind is sound, sounder than mine.

I listen. Everyone is okay. Everything is fine. Good. Now to me. Am I okay? Am I fine? I'm not sure. I'm scared but I don't know why. I know I'm scared because my heart is racing and I want to run away from something terrible and frightening, but nothing is chasing me down except for irrational, horrifying thoughts.

This better not be. It can't be. I won't let it be.

My arm is asleep and parts of my face feel numb. This can't be good. This is something to be scared about. Here's a thought for my fear to grip onto. Now it all makes sense. Why I'm scared. Something awful is happening to my body. What if I'm having a . . . ? I can't say it. The thought sends ice-cold adrenaline surging through my body, jolting me upright. I need to do something about this.

RIGHT NOW.

"9-1-1, what's your emergency?"

"My left arm and face are numb, my heart is racing, and I'm feeling panicky and anxious," I calmly inform the operator.

This better not be. It can't be. I won't let it be.

"Are you breathing okay?" she asks.

"Yes," I reply.

"An ambulance is on the way."

Last night I had a nightmare that I drove off a cliff with Celeste, except that I can't remember if it was actually a nightmare or if I was awake and the thought just randomly—no, *intrusively*—popped into my head. Sometimes I see an image of her drowning in a bathtub.

I feel like I'm drowning. For the past week, each day I've felt my mind sinking deeper and deeper into a dark abyss of crushing waves as I frustratingly attempt to penetrate the surface to no avail. The light at the top is growing dim and the people and things, though right in front of me, are getting harder and harder to see and hear. At any moment I fear I'll just slip away forever. The thought shocks me back to the present for a fleeting moment, for a desperate gasp of air before I grow heavy and begin to descend once more.

This better not be. It can't be. I won't let it be.

If it is, this isn't what it was like the first time. Then, I was anxious, but not this anxious. The heart palpitations terrified me, but I was also sad and angry, really angry. So I meditated, changed my diet, did yoga, and bettered myself. Because it was actually my fault, right? Then, I was just too spoiled and immature to deal with the ultimate sacrifice of motherhood, right? The despair and anguish I felt was something I had to get over by myself by working on myself, which I did and I eventually got better because of it. I triumphed over it. I caused it and I cured it. I was in control all along.

Or so I thought.

If that was the case, then why is it back? Don't say that. It's not back. Everything is okay. Everything is fine. I'm okay. I'm fine. I'm not sad and I'm not angry. I don't have heart palpitations. But I do have chest pain, muscle pain, fatigue, and now, numbness. Those aren't symptoms though, are they? Hard to know when no one talks about it—not my obstetrician, not my midwife, not my family doctor, not anyone at the hospital during labour and delivery.

No, I'm supposed to figure it out while I'm in it. Don't say that; I'm not in it. Everything is okay. Everything is fine. I'm okay. I'm fine. This time, my marriage is solid and my baby sleeps through the night. This time, I'm not overwhelmed. This time I'm happy, euphoric in fact.

This better not be. It can't be. I won't let it be.

So if it's not, then what is it?

"John," I whisper. "John!"

"Yes?" he whispers back.

"I woke up and my arm was numb so I called 9-1-1. The ambulance will be here soon."

He slips out of bed, trying not to wake Eva, and joins me in the hallway.

"You have to stop doing this, Patty," he says. "There are people who really need that ambulance tonight."

Not me. I don't need it. And part of me knows he's right, except my logic is temporarily out of service and anxiety has taken the wheel. Fear is in control. I go back to the master bedroom and change out of my breastfeeding nightgown and into a pair of yoga pants and a T-shirt. I notice how loose my clothes are getting. I've been losing a lot of weight.

The doorbell rings. They're here. I pick up Celeste and rest her head on my left shoulder, which I notice isn't numb anymore. I probably don't need to go to the hospital after all, but if I do end up going, she'll be coming with me. I don't go anywhere without Celeste.

I head down the stairs to the front door and let the paramedics in. We go into the family room, and I sit on the couch as the team of three unfasten their tools. John sits down on the couch next to me. He's calm as calm can be. I'm still anxious even though my numbness is gone and annoyed that I can't calm myself down. We settle in, both knowing what comes next—vitals.

As one paramedic takes my blood pressure, the other takes my temperature and checks my heart rate. I hate having my blood pressure taken. It's a phobia, one of many I have, like flying and snakes. As the cuff gets tighter on my arm and my heart beats ever faster, I tell the paramedic that I have a history of anxiety, that I have white coat syndrome, and that this isn't the first time I've called 9-1-1 for a panic attack, which is probably what this is. I tell him and the other paramedics that I'm sorry for taking up their time and valuable resources and that I'll just make an appointment to see my family doctor first thing in the morning.

"Your blood pressure is high," says the paramedic. "We're looking at stroke or heart attack when it starts getting this high. You need to come with us to the hospital right now."

Well, there's something to say to a person with anxiety. Another shot of adrenaline rushes up through my chest and wraps around my shoulders. I turn to look at John. He shrugs his shoulders. Does that mean he's not sure about whether I have it or whether this could be a life-threatening imminent crisis? I search his face for reassurance.

"Maybe you should go," he says.

Damn. Now I'm petrified.

On the way to the hospital, the paramedic chats with me in the back of the ambulance where I share a black plush-covered bench with him while Celeste is strapped onto the stretcher, still sleeping, so peaceful and oblivious to the urgency unfolding.

I am terrified, but to look at me you wouldn't think so. The paramedic strikes up a conversation about how he doesn't live far and that he jogs up this very hill we're on every single morning. I feign interest and placate him with nods and one-word answers. I figure I can get away with not having to be cordial in this situation since it's possible I could actually be dying in this very moment. You jog? Great. Good for you. I'll just sit over here frozen in fear and wait for the most terrifying event of my life to occur.

This better not be. It can't be. I won't let it be.

We get to the hospital and check in. The nurse asks about my symptoms. I tell her about the numbness and about my history of anxiety. And that's all. I don't venture there . . . yet.

Thankfully, we're given a room with a stretcher to lie on. It's small but it'll do; Celeste is still asleep.

Hours later, I'm given blood tests, and hours after that, the results come in. In the meantime, I've been googling.

Turns out, numbness can be a symptom of it, as can chest pain, intrusive thoughts, a spike in blood pressure, panic attacks, sadness, anger, and something I'd never heard of before called derealization.

The drowning.

The doctor walks in. It's now been six hours.

"Everything looks okay," he informs me. "Everything looks fine."

I'm relieved to hear I'm not at death's door. But if I'm being honest, I know I'm not okay. I know I'm not fine. And I know the onus is on me to say something if I want help.

This better not be. It can't be. I won't let it be.

I look up at the doctor and finally say the words I've been dreading to say out loud.

"I actually have a history of postpartum depression and anxiety," I offer, "and I've been having some of the same symptoms I had a few months after the birth of my first daughter, along with some new ones. I think that's what's happening to me."

The suggestion is shut down. With a wave of his hand in an effort to dismiss my concerns, the doctor smiles and tells me simply not to worry.

"Enjoy motherhood," he counters. "Everything is normal. Just take deep breaths and look at the miracle right in front of you." Looking down at Celeste, his smile grows wider as he takes a deep sigh and says, "They grow up so fast."

BUT THIS IS NOT MOTHERHOOD! I want to yell back. This is postpartum depression and postpartum anxiety and who knows what else. Postpartum obsessive-compulsive disorder? Postpartum bipolar disorder? Postpartum psychosis? These are real maternal mental illnesses that, for the first time, I'm beginning to realize are biological, physical illnesses that require medical attention and not Deepak Chopra.

The doctor senses that his wisdom has not been received well. He offers an olive branch.

"I can schedule an MRI if that would make you feel better," he says. "Numbness can also be a symptom of MS."

"No thanks," I reply. "I'll go see my family doctor tomorrow."

The doctor finishes writing up his report, looks at Celeste, then at me, and says, "Good luck."

The next day I'm prescribed antidepressants. Though I don't score high on the Edinburgh Postpartum Depression Scale because there aren't enough questions about postpartum anxiety, given my history, my family doctor is pretty sure that's what we're dealing with. I ask for therapy, but since there aren't any good psychiatrists in the area, according to my doctor, I'll have to go without and rely solely on medication to help me through.

Tears flow as I swallow my first pill. Within a few weeks, I'll start to feel better. Within a few months, I'll feel the best I've ever felt in my entire life, and I'll begin to question why I wasn't ever screened, assessed, and treated for maternal mental illness during either of my pregnancies and postpartum; why I wasn't ever screened, assessed, and treated for anxiety as a child; why I wasn't ever screened, assessed, and treated for depression as an adolescent; why I wasn't ever screened, assessed, and treated for panic disorder as a young adult; and why, unless I ask for it, I probably won't be screened, assessed, and treated for a mental illness going forward. After all, I've still got menopause to contend with.

More than question, I'll begin to write about it and connect with researchers and advocates across the country. I'll become an advocate myself and participate in rallies to demand political change because it's unfathomable to me that women in Canada still aren't being properly screened, assessed, and treated for maternal mental illnesses.

This better not be. It can't be. I won't let it be.

Patricia Tomasi is a journalist, an advocate, and a mom of two. She writes for *Huffington Post Canada,* focusing primarily on maternal mental health after suffering from perinatal depression, perinatal anxiety, and perinatal bipolar disorder— twice. Patricia believes Canada needs a national maternal mental health strategy that includes universal screening for all perinatal mood and anxiety disorders.

DO YOU WANT DINNER?

Michael Landsberg

IF ANY OF YOU FEEL *let down by this story, I will buy you dinner. So far no one has ever tried to cash in on that.*

"I know you struggled with depression in the nineties, but I've never heard you speak about it. I've only read about your journey. Would it be okay if I ask you how you're doing in the interview?" I ask two-time Stanley Cup–winning hockey player Stéphane Richer as we walk out of the green room right before we go on to film an episode of TSN's *Off the Record*.

He hesitates.

I continue on and say, "I don't want to embarrass you. You don't owe me anything, but I thought it would be interesting. And, if it is okay with you, I will share about my own struggles."

His eyes widen, and he turns to face me. "You struggle?" he asks, surprised.

"Oh yeah," I say with conviction. "As a matter of fact, I just came out of my year-and-a-half-long biggest struggle ever."

We go on set and start to film. The interview is going well. Before our air time runs out and we go to a commercial break, I say, "I know you've struggled with depression. How bad was it? And how are you doing now?"

He responds, "Well, it was bad enough that I tried to take my life five days after winning the Stanley Cup."

I thank him and share that I, too, have struggled—I'm not ashamed; I'm not embarrassed. It's just something that I have experienced, and it's horrible—but that doesn't mean I'm trying to bury it.

We go to commercial break, and I don't give it another thought. But the next day I start getting emails—twenty-two of them, actually. Twenty of them are from men, and they all say the same thing: Hey, Michael, I'm telling you something I've never told another human being. I'm telling you because I just watched both you and Stéphane Richer openly share your struggles with depression. I've never seen two men who seem to have it reasonably together, who are successful, talk about suffering from a mental illness without shame or embarrassment, or sounding weak. But now I have, and because of that, I'm going to share my story with you.

I correspond with all of these people, and I make the point that if they've shared with me, then the next step is to share their stories with someone else and to go get help.

I am now super pissed-off at myself that I didn't talk about my mental health earlier. With this interview, I discover the power of sharing. I confirm that, yes, I suffer from depression, I'm on medication, I'm not embarrassed, and I know that this mental illness is a physical illness in my brain. Just by saying that, a person can change other people's lives.

One of the people who was apparently watching that day is a guy named Tyson Williams of North Battleford, Saskatchewan. He sends me an email, and I send him one back. He writes, Good for you and Stéphane, but it's probably too late for me because I'm too shy. This is too painful for me, I'm never going to share, but good for you. I know you will help others. I've struggled for too long. I can't see myself ever going to see a doctor.

We email back and forth, and the last thing I write is, Dude, you're suffering and you're in pain. What do you have to lose? What could be worse than where you are right now? He answers, Maybe I'll think about it.

A year and a half later, I get an email. It says, Dear Michael, you won't remember me; it's Tyson Williams from North Battleford, Saskatchewan. But I do remember him. He continues, You and I exchanged emails a year and a half ago, and what you don't know is that I wasn't completely truthful—I was much worse than I had said. I was actually in my closet with a belt around my neck, and I was in the process of ending my life when I heard the computer chime. I thought that maybe it was someone in my family, so I went to the computer and it was you responding to my email. I was shocked because I didn't think that people on television would respond to emails from guys like me, but you and I corresponded five times—and after each of the first four emails, I went back to the closet to finish the job. I had written notes to my family, I had decided I was going to end it, but the last thing you said to me resonated with me. You didn't know the stakes you were playing with, but you said I had nothing to lose if I went to get help, so the next day I went to my family doctor and here we are a year and a half later and I feel good about myself. I feel great about my life. I'm better than I ever was in my life. All because two guys on TV opened up and publicly shared their personal struggles with depression.

You want a dinner?

Okay, because I'm not done yet. A couple of summers ago, I am asked to go to Saskatoon, and if you know your Saskatchewan geography—and I imagine you don't—North Battleford is about a ninety-minute drive from Saskatoon. Canadian hockey coach Mike Babcock has a fundraiser for mental health, and he asks me to come and be the emcee, and of course I think, *Oh my God, Mike Babcock is asking me. This is so cool! I'm going to be standing on stage looking down at Mike Babcock, and I can make fun of him! I own his ass for two hours! Oh yeah!*

I ask if I can bring a guest, and they say yes. I write Tyson Williams and ask if he wants to be my guest at this amazing event.

He replies, Oh I would love to do that but there would be no way. I would be too uncomfortable. I'm too shy; it's just not me.

I write back, Come on, dude. You're with me. I'm the friggin' emcee for God's sake. I got your back!

He replies again, No, I can't do it.

So, I persist. Well, you could bring your fiancée.

Okay, he finally agrees.

By the way, some time after the original situation, he sends me an email with a picture of himself in a Boston Bruins jersey, holding a baby. The baby is in a Bruins sleeper, and the caption reads, THIS IS WHAT HAPPENS WHEN YOU SHARE.

This is a picture of his newborn baby daughter.

I tell Tyson that the event is going to be great. Tons of celebrities will be there. It's a thousand dollars a person. There will probably be at least five hundred people there; this is how important it is to this community. I tell him that it's going to be a big deal and to just prepare for it.

He shows up. I can see him walking toward me. I know it's him, first of all, because I have seen pictures of him, but second of all, because he is wearing cargo shorts and a T-shirt, which is so charming. This guy doesn't understand, and he certainly doesn't care. He is just like, "this is me." What shocks me is that his fiancée is dressed beautifully, and I say to her, "Hello? You didn't think to get dressed together and maybe mention, 'Hello, Honey, I'm wearing a nice dress and you're dressed in cargo shorts?'" (Which, by the way, is the lowest form of clothing that anyone can wear out of the house besides sweatpants.)

I get up on the stage and I say, "The reason I'm here today dates back to October 24, 2009, when I shared my mental health struggles for the first time on TV. One particular person watching that day was Tyson Williams." I proceed to share what happened that day when Tyson and I emailed back and forth, and then I tell the audience, "Tyson is here today. I'd like you to stand up, Tyson."

He sheepishly stands up. You can see his head is down and he is looking at the floor, and all of a sudden everybody stands up. And everyone is cheering him. Mike Babcock and all of these hockey stars that he has watched all of his life are twenty feet away from him—and they are all cheering *him*. And it lasts for about a minute, and I am on the stage thinking, *Wow, life is pretty wild.* When you think of Tyson Williams in his closet with a belt around his neck ready to end his life, and here he is being cheered at this event, for this cause, his fiancée at his side and a baby daughter at home, and I think, *This is the coolest thing!*

So, do you want dinner? . . . I'm not done.

I'll just give you one more layer to this story. Last May, I got an email from Tyson and it says, Hey Michael, don't be mad at me . . . but would you be the best man at my wedding?

I message him right away. Like yeah. I'd love to.

Last September, I travel half an hour north of Prince Albert. I am thinking, *Could you find a farther place for me to go?* So here I am at this event in his community, without a single soul I would know, standing at the front of the community centre, wearing a suit while everyone else is wearing Saskatchewan Roughriders jerseys. (He told me I had to wear a suit! I don't wear suits, but I did this special favour for him, so I wanted to scream out, *This is wrong, people! Wrong!*)

I'm standing up there and Tyson's fiancée is walking down the aisle, and he greets her. We're on the stage and his daughter, who is now a couple of years old, runs toward him and he picks her up. So it's Tyson and his soon-to-be wife, their daughter, whoever is presiding over the service, a couple of other family members, and me. And that's when I think, *Life's REALLY messed up . . . and incredible.*

Because of that, and since then, I have discovered that the most impactful thing I can do is simply talk about my experiences and let others know that if they suffer from mental illness, they are not alone.

I start an organization, a community, an online movement called SickNotWeak, dedicated to just that—talking and letting people know that they aren't alone. Little did I know almost ten years ago that saying something so off the cuff could make a difference not only in my life but in the lives of so many others.

One of the best-known personalities in Canadian broadcasting, Michael Landsberg was the host of TSN's *Off the Record*, a television sports talk show that ran for eighteen seasons. An ambassador for Bell Let's Talk, Michael was named one of the Canadian Alliance on Mental Illness and Mental Health's Champions of Mental Health, as well as one of CAMH's 150

Difference Makers. Landsberg is the founder of SickNotWeak, a non-profit organization and an online community where people living with mental illness can share stories, encouragement, and support. For his longstanding dedication to promoting mental health awareness, Landsberg was honoured with the Humanitarian Award at the Canadian Screen Awards. Today, he hosts *Landsberg in the Morning* on TSN Radio.

THE QUESTION

Enza Tiberi-Checchia

I GO OUTSIDE TO MAKE a very important call to a spiritual psycho-therapist to have a "discovery session." It is a beautiful summer day, the sun shining on my face and Mother Earth beneath my feet.

I dial the number. The voice on the other end answers, "Good morning, Enza. The intention for this call is for each of us to determine if it is a good fit for us to work together. Can you tell me your story?"

"Well," I begin, "I have experienced over six major depressive episodes since 1988, my last one being eight years ago. I have been off medication for almost a year now, and I would like to work with you so I do not sink into depression ever again."

I continue, matter-of-factly. "Immediately following my first major psychotic break in 1988, I was three months pregnant with my first child and my father, only fifty years old, died by suicide."

I continue the recount like an unbiased news reporter. "The day before we laid my father to rest, I received doctor's orders for three weeks of bedrest because I was in danger of miscarrying my child. The day before I was to return to work, a termination letter from my employer was delivered to my door by a cab driver, and a couple of weeks after that my house was broken into."

There is a generous pause before the therapist breaks the intensity with her response. "These are deeply traumatic experiences for any human being to process, and they all happened to you within a short, six-month period. How did you process them at the time or get through them since then?"

My answer is simple, yet profound. "I just keep going."

There is a shift and opening in my consciousness as I hear myself say those words: I just keep going.

It's as if every fibre of my being recognizes for the very first time that maybe mental illness is not who I am. Maybe it is actually just something that I experience as a result of untreated, unprocessed trauma. This liberates and unshackles my deepest fear that mental illness is a life sentence, my life sentence. I realize parole is not just possible, but probable!

It invites me onto a path of self-discovery and awareness that empowers and supports me to learn how to regulate my emotions and rewire my brain. I learn to live an authentic, balanced, and joy-filled life, making me unrecognizable to myself.

I continue to heal from the traumatic experiences in my life, and I also excavate the gifts that come from them—the skills and abilities I developed as a result of my strategy to "just keep going" are evaluated and upgraded, transformed, or repurposed as required to serve me today.

In the still, quiet moments between therapy sessions, I hear the following words, and it occurs to me that they represent a public charge that needs to be shared:

Change is not for the faint of heart;
Choose instead to follow your heart.

No longer keep the silence;
Know that silence is the violence.

Speak to be heard;
Sometimes disrupt and disturb.

Know there is hope;
Provide a new scope.

Honour your call;
You will not fall.

There's a world to rearrange;
You are the change.

A week later, I find myself addressing over seven hundred and fifty people at a gala, Hatsquerade, an annual fundraising event for Hats On For Awareness, a charity I have co-founded with my dear friend and colleague, Benny Caringi. The journey to this point seems almost surreal. I stand, shaking as I make my declaration and speak these words, "I will lead the charge to change how we see and treat mental illness. My life experiences with mental illness led me to the path of my life's work. I face that path with gratitude, honour, and great privilege, for through the grace that has brought me here, there is much to share, much to improve, much to inspire, and much to ignite."

I leave the stage, and with a big gulp, I summon my conscious business coach and ask, "Now what?" With her help, I find the words that form Mi Vision and Mi Message and the courage to share them via Mi Etcetera—the platform from which I advocate and speak for those without a voice. I am deeply grateful to find my life's purpose. I will never give up hope for the end of suffering for those who are struggling with mental illness. My quest to support myself led me to my life's work, and along the way, I have reclaimed everything I require to live a purposeful life. It is hard to believe it all started with one revolutionary question: How do you process trauma?

"Mental illness did not break me, it broke me open." Chief visionary officer and co-founder of Hats On For Awareness and founder of Mi Etcetera, Enza Tiberi-Checchia is a passionate mental health advocate, philanthropist, speaker, and blogger. She resides in Mississauga, Ontario. To learn more about Enza's work, please visit mietcetera.com.

WORDS

Katherine Hambleton

IT HAPPENS SO FAST, TOO fast. The front door explodes. "Get in the back room," one of the three men snarls, guns pointed at us.

Heart is pounding, senses are heightened. Amygdala switches on, and the adrenaline begins to surge. No time to think. No time to process. No time to hesitate. My four friends and I follow this command and corral into the back room upstairs. As he closes the door, he barks, "Don't move."

We don't.

"Stay where you are," he orders.

We comply.

"Don't do anything stupid." He looks at me—his gaze running right through me—shaking me to the core. He extends his weapon toward me; gun pressed against the side of my head, my heart is full of fear.

There is an awkward silence that seems long, too long. We hear the commotion in the other room. Mind is racing. *What is happening? How did I find myself here? Will I die?*

I am too young to die, I think.

I am only fifteen years old, living with my older sister in a rental property that my father manages. I help my sister with her own young daughter while she works and goes to school. We just recently had new tenants move into the second house on the property—where I am now, sitting captive at gunpoint. The renters are a young couple, and I have made quick friends with the woman, who isn't that much older than I. They are sleeping in the other bedroom. At least they were . . .

The uncomfortable silence in the room is replaced with detonating fear. The door swings open. One of the accomplices carries the woman, my friend, into the room. Wounded and seizing, she vomits up paint. The man keeping us hostage is visibly shaken. He backs up. "Help her," he instructs.

He watches as I do what I can. Her seizure finally subsiding, I place her onto her side in the recovery position. She keeps throwing up. *Please don't die*, I think. Thankfully she doesn't.

"Stay there. Don't you dare move," our captor says as he backs out of the room, closing the door behind him.

A deafening silence ensues. I don't know for how long, but eventually we emerge from the room, blood and paint everywhere—a horror version of a Jackson Pollock painting.

"I am going to my house," I tell the others as I run home. My sister is there.

"What happened to you?" she asks. There is no time for long explanations. She calls 9-1-1, then our father.

My father arrives. I am still shaken, longing for comforting words like a child seeking approval, reassurance. I need him to embrace me, ask me how I am, what happened, if I will be all right. But instead, the real trauma begins.

Alternatively the words—aggressive, angry, and accusatory— fly out of his mouth. "What the f--- were you doing there?"

Words: indelible, irreversible, and intolerable. At this moment, I wish to be back in that room, with my friends, knowing that I am not alone; preferable to these utterances from someone who is supposed to love me. Instead, I am barraged with judgment and blame.

I spiral. To be fair, I was already spinning. I have a mountain of adverse childhood experiences that have held me, leading me into a world of addiction and self-sabotaging behaviours. But now—now the downward trajectory deepens and quickens with a new urgency. A new set of labels attach themselves to me: dropout, runaway, street kid, drug user—*crystal meth addict*.

One night, while working in an after-hours rave club, it hits me—the realization that I know too much. Street knowledge can be dangerous, and it occurs to me that I need to leave. I run again. This time I end up back home, slowly trading in my dangerous addictions for obsession with achievement. I go back to high school, go to college, work hard to fill the void with good grades, awards, and scholarships. But I don't give up all my vices: I still occasionally partake in the sweet numbing effects of drugs and alcohol.

While in my final year of high school, a friend and I are out drinking on St. Patrick's Day, and we have had more than we should.

"I am okay to drive," my friend announces.

"Um, no you aren't," I slur. "Let's call a cab."

"Really?"

We are at the car, and we get in.

"I have to go to the bathroom," my friend mutters.

Great, I think as I scooch into the driver's seat, key in ignition. I know I won't be driving home because I can't drive standard. But at least my friend won't be able to drive either if I am in the front seat, and we can stay warm as we wait for a taxi.

Knock, knock. My brow furrows in confusion as I roll down the window. "Hi Officer," I say.

Care and control charge. Me at the police station. I stagger into one of my morning classes, hours later, still stinking of booze. The irony sinks in, the aha moment seeping into me on a cellular level. It is time. It is time for me to face the words: the words of my father, the words of my abusers, and the strongest words of all—the words in my own head.

I kiss my young daughter's head. "I love you, little one," I say. "See you soon."

I've put in quite a long week working many shifts at the hospital and teaching. I am a registered nurse. I haven't fully conquered that urge to constantly achieve, but I am getting better. I drive to my Wings of Change meeting.

"Welcome, everyone," I begin, going over the usual housekeeping items: coffee, water, washrooms, etc.

We go around the room introducing ourselves. "Hi, my name is Katherine," I continue. "I am the program administrator for Wings of Change Peer Support and the facilitator for this chapter. I've been working in health care for fifteen years now . . ."

The meeting continues, and we go through our readings, setting the expectations before we discuss the evening's topics. Our chapter is one of more than twenty across the nation, founded by Natalie Harris, a paramedic who suffered an operational stress injury. In two short years, it has grown from one little chapter in her hometown to a thriving national group, revolutionizing peer support and the mental health culture for those working in the circle of care. It is a group for our community heroes: first responders, law enforcement personnel, health care providers, communications officers, animal workers, funeral directors, child protection, and judiciary services—just to name a few.

I have been in this role for over a year now, overseeing the operations of the organization. I provide online peer knowledge exchanges, relevant resources, social media presence, and support for existing and new groups. I have been a mental health advocate for a while now, and sliding into this position has been both comforting and gratifying.

As the evening unfolds, we share words: positive and supportive words, edifying words. Words that build one another up, provide comfort and solace.

I realize in this moment just how powerful words can be. They can tear us down, but they can also save us. We are all really still children, looking for approval, for comfort . . . for reassurance.

As I leave the meeting, I am grateful for Wings of Change and the opportunity I have to be a part of something that can help so many people. The best way for me to heal and combat all the hurtful words that have pierced my own soul is to fill the world with greater words, healing words: words that can change for the better. And with this knowledge, I drive home to my daughter, embracing her as I walk through the door. "Hello, my beautiful *menina*. I love you to the sun and back."

Katherine Hambleton is a mother, a wife, and a registered nurse. She achieved diplomas of health sciences in nursing and paramedicine, holding a speciality in emergency nursing and a certificate in critical care. She is the program administrator for Wings of Change Peer Support, a support group established for first responders and other community heroes. Through both personal and professional adversities in her life, Katherine has been a dedicated advocate for first responder wellness.

BETTER

Stéphane Grenier with Jim Davis

I CATCH PART OF AN interview on CBC Radio's *Ottawa Morning* show. Host Robyn Bresnahan sets up the segment. "Hill staffers have high-pressure jobs and long hours, and earlier this year that job caught up with Paul Wernick . . . He wound up in hospital after trying to take his own life . . ."

I listen as the young staffer shares his story. "Again, we live in a society, especially on the Hill, where there is a kind of tough it out, drink to feel better, road warrior, take whatever comes at me . . ."

The interview continues, and MP Charlie Angus follows, expressing concern about improving the culture and services in the Canadian government workplace, making sure that the chasm between workplace support and medical mental health services is narrowed.

I can't help but think, *This is no better or worse than most Canadian workplaces I consult with.* However, it happens to be the nation's capital, Parliament Hill, the head of our country, which, as a workplace, needs to change. But change is slow and laboured in most organizations. It is a struggle and tiring, like pushing wet noodles uphill: Every. Single. Day. It is a grind.

I look at a news release from the Governor General's office: I have been appointed as a Member to the Order of Canada, an award that, according to its website, recognizes distinguished service in or to a particular community, group, or field of activity. The motto is *Desiderantes Meliorem Patriam*, which translates to "They desire a better country." I read the single sentence that is supposed to sum up a lifetime of work:

Stéphane Grenier, C.M., M.S.C., C.D., LL.D.
Val-des-Monts, Quebec

For his leadership in mental health advocacy and programming for the military and general public, notably as founding president of Mental Health Innovations.

Although I am very honoured and grateful, I am struck by the duplicity of the situation. While I am not a negative person, I am a realist. The very government that will bestow this distinction upon me for my efforts in workplace mental health is the same government that needs to also work on improving its own mental health culture. Most workplaces need to implement what I advocate for: strong, sustainable, and credible mental health programs to complement the current system.

Back in 2007, I received the Meritorious Service Cross. I remember sitting in Rideau Hall, listening to Governor General Michaëlle Jean's speech: "Some of you have developed programs designed to help Canadian Forces' members and their families . . . All of your accomplishments show the depth of your commitment. They are also reminders of how our military has changed to keep pace with our evolving society."

Cocktails followed—congratulatory slaps on the back, handshakes, and photo ops. Despite all this hoopla and fanfare, there was the probability that things would just "continue to be" if I did not carry on advocating. I knew that if I wanted to see reform on a revolutionary scale, the effort would be relentless. And I was right. The next week—the next day, even—I found myself again justifying and defending mental health initiatives to some of the very same people who had congratulated me at the ceremony.

My mind wanders back to when I returned from my tour in Rwanda, to when I first noticed changes in myself, changes that I would later learn were connected to my PTSD. I received a call from the military logistic staff: "Your equipment from Rwanda has arrived in Ottawa," the voice on the other end of the line informed me.

I promptly drove to the airport, signed for my equipment, and brought it home. The following weekend was unusually sunny and warm for April, so I decided to open up my barracks boxes and equipment bags, and clean and sort through things in the driveway. As I began my work, my young daughter, Véronique, was happily taking advantage of the good weather, riding her tricycle around on our dead-end street. "*Regarde-moi, papa!*" she chirped as she pedalled back and forth.

After watching her enjoy herself for a few minutes, I opened everything up, attached the hose, and started by cleaning my boots. I picked one up and began spraying the sole, which still had Rwandan soil stuck in it. As the water rolled away from the boot, a reddish tint bled down the driveway. Red: the stain of blood, the hue of rage, and the naturally occurring pigment of Rwandan earth.

I had seen my first war-torn human corpse without warning on that tour. Because of the weather conditions and time of day, I couldn't tell for sure if it was a man or a woman: the body just lay there by the side of the road like a piece of unwanted garbage someone had pitched from their vehicle. The limbs looked dislocated and mangled, and it was obvious the person had met a sudden, violent death. This was the first of thousands of corpses I would see during my ten-month tour, including a little girl, on her belly, with her arms tucked close to her body and her fists near her head, which was turned slightly to one side in a posture Véronique often assumed while lying in bed.

Of course, I had seen dead people before. Like most adults, I had been to a funeral and had watched war movies and documentaries about the Holocaust. But seeing actual bodies in a conflict setting made the shock of death hit home in an eerily visceral way. My mind now associated the soil's redness with blood, which imparted its own shade of distaste all over the ground.

Véronique became curious by all the military gear. She started walking up the driveway to see what I was doing. With the juxtaposition of these two sights, I panicked. The idea of my daughter and the Rwandan soil being in close proximity—two opposing worlds about to collide—sent me into an uncontrollable ball of urgency. I could not let the soil—the *dirt* of a country that had been extremely cruel to itself, the red earth, a symbol associated with the human cruelty I had witnessed in Rwanda— touch my daughter.

I swore under my breath, and then a little too briskly I yelled, "*Ne touche pas ça. Éloigne-toi de là.*"

I then instructed her, more gruffly than I liked, to get back on her tricycle and go up to the house.

To anyone who may have walked by, the scene would have appeared just like a father having a bad day, but to me, inside, it felt as if I was completely coming undone. Normally I could process strong emotions and moderate my reaction. My outside voice could be monitored and didn't have to match my inside voice. However, now, it felt as if the filter I once possessed had disappeared, and I had no idea how to find it again. I felt as though I had no control over my reaction that day. The old me would have distracted Véronique and simply said, "Look at the squirrel," or picked her up gently, redirecting her.

This was the beginning of a long journey that would span decades. I continued on, faced with my own undiagnosed post-traumatic stress and took a personal interest in the way the Canadian Forces dealt with mental health issues. I coined the term "operational stress injury" (OSI) and conceived, developed, implemented, and managed a government-based peer support program for the Canadian military. After retiring, I created Mental Health Innovations, a social enterprise dedicated to developing non-clinical mental health interventions as a complement to traditional clinical care. And I wrote an autobiography, *After the War: Surviving PTSD and Changing Mental Health Culture*, to awaken the nation to the toll that moral conflict and stress injuries are taking on Canadians.

I go to my computer and open my email to reread a letter from Jim Davis, a man whose son fell in Afghanistan:

Dear Stéphane,

I just finished reading your book. Stéph, you travelled to hell and back. I truly believe that God took you there and brought you safely home so you could tell us what hell on earth is like and help others survive the experience.

I now know that if my boy survived, he would have come home with a horrible operational stress injury. There is a passage in your book that reminds me of something he said to me: It was Jan 23, 2006 (he had been in the military for ten years and did a tour in Bosnia), and he and I took a walk in the snow just before he boarded his plane to Afghanistan. He said, "Dad, there is something that really bothers me."

I said, "What, Paul?"

"I don't think I can kill a man," he answered.

Stéphane, I am sure that he would have returned home with a horrible OSI caused by his moral conflict.

Your story has helped me a lot. From what I have learned of that moment in Afghanistan, my son was spared that horrible task. In his final minutes of his life, he had his gun pointed on the taxi driver and asked for the command to fire. Being true Canadian soldiers, the order was not given in the hopes the taxi would change direction.

My son did not kill anyone.

Thank you, Stéphane, for writing your book.

Your friend,

Jim

This kind of feedback—in addition to bearing witness to true, lasting, and concrete change—is more important than any possible commendation. To begin with, I just wanted a better employer for myself and for those who also experience operational stress injuries. When you push to make the country a better place for one, ironically, you make it a better place for everyone: *Desiderantes Meliorem Patriam*, indeed.

Stéphane Grenier is a mental health innovator, advocate, speaker, and entrepreneur. He retired from the Canadian military as a lieutenant colonel after serving twenty-nine years. In 2012, he retired from the military and created Mental Health Innovations (MHI), a social enterprise dedicated to developing non-clinical mental health interventions as a complement to traditional clinical care. His autobiography, *After the War: Surviving PTSD and Changing Mental Health Culture,* was published by University of Regina Press. To learn more about Stéphane Grenier and his work, please visit stephanegrenier.com.

RESOURCES

Please note that these resources were available at time of publication. However, Wintertickle Press cannot take responsibility if these resources become unavailable. If you are in crisis, please seek out medical attention immediately.

CANADA

- Crisis Services Canada
  Toll-free crisis line: 1-833-456-4566
  TEXT 45645
  Chat http://www.crisisservicescanada.ca

- Kids Help Phone Ages 5-20; 1-800-668-6868

USA

- National Suicide Prevention Lifeline: 1-800-273-8255
- The Crisis Text Line (crisistextline.org) is the only 24/7 nationwide crisis-intervention text-message hotline. The Crisis Text Line can be reached by texting HOME to 741-741.

UNITED KINGDOM

- Samaritans.org: 116 (UK)

LIST OF CONTRIBUTORS

Heidi Allen

Marleah Atlookan

Autumn Aurelia

Karen Copeland

V.N. Doran

Heather Down

Jeff Emmerson

H.A. Fraser

Terri Lynn Futcher

Serge Gagné

Stéphane Grenier (with Jim Davis)

Tim Grutzius

Katherine Hambleton

Natalie Harris

Asante Haughton

Matthew Heneghan

L.A. Hill

Zach Hofer

Julie Jolicoeur

Catherine Kenwell

Michael Landsberg

Kate Lyon Osher

Jorden Mathias

Sarah Beth McClure

Deb McGrath

Diane McKay

Christine Newman

Glen Oliver

Amber Phillips

Zoey Raffay

Maud Revel

Michelle Sertage

April Shaw

Reema Sukumaran

Courtney Taylor

Ann Thomas

Enza Tiberi-Checchia

Patricia Tomasi

Jodie Toresdahl

Javier Vargas

CONNECT

Do you have a story to share? If you would like your story to be considered for future editions of *Brainstorm Revolution*, please email your story idea to brainstormsubmissions@hotmail.com. Be sure to follow Wintertickle Press on social media!

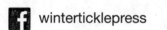 wintericklepress 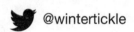 @wintertickle